BREAST CANCER

One Illness, Two Women, Four Seasons

BREAST CANCER

One Illness, Two Women, Four Seasons

MARY ELLEN HAVARD

MARY OPENLANDER, P.T.

PENULTIMATE PUBLISHING
ST. LOUIS, MISSOURI

Publisher: PenUltimate Publishing
Design/Production: Renée Duenow
Cover and Section Opener Illustrations: Joanne Kluba
Printer: BookMasters, Inc.

©2005 by PenUltimate Publishing

606 North and South Road
Saint Louis, Missouri   63130
Phone: (314) 862-3842
Fax: (314) 862-5911
E-mail: penultim@swbell.net
Website: www.penultimatepbl.com

Library of Congress Control Number: 2004096420

Havard, Mary Ellen, 1942
Openlander, Mary, 1954
Breast cancer: one illness, two women, four seasons/Mary Ellen Havard and Mary Openlander
p. cm.
ISBN 0-9760675-0-1
1. Health   2. Breast Cancer   3. Trager

Printed in the United States
Printing 10 9 8 7 6 5 4 3 2

The authors gratefully acknowledge permission to quote from the following published work:
Louise L. Hay. *Wisdom Cards* ©2000 Hay House, Inc: Carlsbad, CA.
Reprinted by permission of Hay House.

The authors gratefully acknowledge permission to reproduce copyright poems by Jan Newhouse:
Directions ©2000. Reprinted by permission of the author.
Into the Valley of the Shadow ©2000. Reprinted by permission of the author.
Thanksgiving ©2001. Reprinted by permission of the author.

The authors gratefully acknowledge permission to reproduce the photograph of the sculpture
Cradling Her Sorrow by Nancy Fried.

Ginny Guyol McShane
Grace Middleton Havard
Mary Gumble Levy
Copper Finnegan Olivos
Ellen Waldbart Ellis
Karen Cohen Towerman

These are women I love dearly. I share the disease cancer with them,
and it took them from me long before I was ready to let them go.
To each of them I dedicate this book.

MARY ELLEN HAVARD

For my husband, Patrick,
and sons, Michael and Denis,
with all my love.

MARY OPENLANDER

ACKNOWLEDGMENTS

*B*ehind every entry in this journal is a group of people whose support
and strength were there for me and for whom I am deeply grateful.

*My wonderful husband, whose love has given me my voice; my son,
Mark, whose love for me, concern and compassion were so much more
than he was able to put into words; my son, Michael, who suffered in so
many ways because of my illness; and the other members of "my team":*

*My family; friends; neighbors; the parish of Christ the King, who cared
for me, fed our family, and watched over us; and the prayer groups who
held us up each and every day.*

*Dr. Peter Weiss, Dr. Jerome Levy, Dr. Patrick Openlander, Dr. Carlos Perez,
Dr. Marie Taylor, Angie Creg, Allison Smith, Linda Iliff, Jill Bokern,
Elaine Muellerleile, Mimi Butler, and Kathleen Lane.*

*Mia Fitzgerald; the staff at Cedar Creek Conference Center; Eleanor
and Dan Ferry, who generously provided Mary and me the peace
and beauty of the country in which to put our two journals together;
and Mary James and Julie Woodward for their photographs.*

*My brothers and sisters—Catherine, John, Bob, Joe, and Rita, and their
families. Your love and support are always there for me.*

*My dear friend Winnie Sullivan and all at PenUltimate for their patient
guidance and encouragement.*

*But especially Mary, whose hands and touch brought back my sense
of wholeness and got me back into my dancing shoes!*

MARY ELLEN HAVARD

This book is the result of a long-held desire of mine to write something about this wonderful work, the *Trager*® Approach. I am grateful to all my teachers over the years: Dr. Milton Trager, Gary Brownlee, Carol Campbell, Betty Fuller, Cathy Hammond, Jean Hopkins, Deane Juhan, Gail Stewart, Roger Tolle, and tutors and practitioners too numerous to name. I am especially grateful to the small contingent of *Trager* folks in St. Louis—Mary Laffey Adams, Mike Elliff, Susan Kissinger, and Jenn Tara Ward—for all the fun and inspiration we have shared that has helped keep this work alive and developing for me. To those clients, especially early in my training, who were so open and interested in *Trager*—you were the clay in my hands, and mentored me in a way no professional teacher could.

As I wrote I relied on a variety of people for information and feedback. I'd like to thank Jane Kraus, RN, for clarifying details of the practice of medical oncology; Winnie Sullivan, of PenUltimate Publishing, for her patient attention to questions and clear, thorough answers in addition to having suggested that our journal could be a book; Judy Roos, at PenUltimate, for her invaluable input to the process, and Renée Duenow for complementing the book's content with her imaginative design; Henry Bornstein for his editorial help and advice in describing the *Trager* Approach; Denis Openlander for reminding me, from the university student's perspective, what makes good writing; my coauthor Mary Ellen Havard for holding high the value of writing with heart and for being so willing, on so many levels and in so many ways. Additionally, the curiosity and suggestions of family and friends— especially my parents, Robert and Teresa O'Connor—truly fed the process of writing. Thank you for your steadfastness. I love you dearly.

Photographs of Mary Ellen and me practicing *Trager* are courtesy of my son Michael, who captured my love of the work through his lens. Thank you, Michael.

Finally, I am deeply grateful to my husband and dear friend, Patrick, for being my biggest supporter over the years. His early and deep appreciation of the *Trager* Approach helped spur me on. His tireless listening and shared in-depth knowledge of the body/mind connection has deepened my understanding and development not only in the *Trager* Approach but also in healing in general. Thank you from the bottom of my heart.

MARY OPENLANDER

FOREWORD

Breast cancer affects nearly 200,000 women in the United States every year. Though therapeutic modalities have been able to successfully treat—and even cure—this disease, in a growing number of cases early detection is still key to longevity. Educating people about breast cancer in general, stressing the importance of screening, and raising the awareness of symptoms are steps necessary to improving care.

As a medical oncologist, I have been privileged to lead many patients and their families through the diagnosis, treatment, and outcome of breast cancer. During this journey, I particularly emphasize the "positives" of having cancer—the sudden realization of "what is truly important," the deepening and strengthening of relationships, the spiritual awakening—that can act as a guide and enable patients to endure the emotional and physical stress of treatment.

Throughout, it is the people who offer support—family, friends, physicians, therapists—who are so vital to the healing process. Knowing this, Mary Ellen assembled her team, including the unique talents of Mary, a *Trager* therapist, to help her survive the first year. Together, they give a strikingly honest account of a woman's breast cancer experience —capturing the fears, emotional trials, and physical changes associated with the disease and its treatment.

As a medical practitioner, I found this book able to portray both the sensitivities and the insensitivities of our health care system. This is an important read for all health care professionals, including medical and nursing students, patients with (or with a history of) breast cancer, family members of cancer patients, and meditative, massage and physical therapists. As this book shows, breast cancer treatment is more than chemotherapy, radiation, and statistics: it is the story of an individual and her personal journey toward healing.

PETER D. WEISS, M.D.

CONTENTS

INTRODUCTION

*W*hen I was told I had breast cancer, my world flew apart. I was pulled in opposing directions, living in two worlds. There was the one of curling up in a ball and crying, refusing to eat, refusing to sleep, refusing to think. There was the other of facing the issues and making a plan. I had a job to do, and that job was called survival. During my treatment I lived partly in one world and partly in the other. For some of the time, I collapsed in a heap. And this, in turn, gave me the strength to get on with it.

The doctors told me that I was facing a difficult year and that the treatments they outlined for me would be rigorous. My first inclination was to run out of their offices screaming. I felt as if I were standing before my house, watching it burn to the ground, while people talked to me of their plans for retrieving my belongings inside. How could all the medical experts be taking their sweet time making elaborate plans, while I was consumed with urgency, watching everything go up in flames? I didn't want to waste a minute putting the thing out!

I asked Mary Openlander, a physical therapist and Trager practitioner, to help me. Mary had never given a series of Trager sessions to someone actively undergoing cancer treatment. She was used to seeing these patients after they had finished treatment. She was confident, though, that her work would provide the emotional and physical support that I wanted. Mary was also interested in learning more about the needs of cancer patients and the role of a Trager practitioner in assisting these patients in the healing process.

Because of her desire to learn, Mary suggested that we each keep a journal, recording our impressions and experiences during this time. I agreed. I was so relieved that Mary thought I would live long enough to finish the treatments! Thus, writing became part of my healing. And the journal entries, written as they were lived, reflect the personal and physical challenges, the fears, uncertainties, and realizations that filled these days.

After recording our thoughts and impressions for more than a year, Mary and I shared our writing with one another. Gradually, our separate entries melded into this book. Now, extending an invitation to come along on our journey, we share them with you.

MARY ELLEN HAVARD
MARY OPENLANDER

BREAST CANCER

One Illness, Two Women, Four Seasons

Spring

Today I found out that it is likely that I have breast cancer. I parked the car some distance from the doctor's office because it was such a beautiful day and I felt like walking. I even talked to myself about how well I felt and how much energy I have. I could tell by the look on my doctor's face during my examination that she was alarmed. She arranged for me to take my last year's mammogram with me to another facility where I had a diagnostic mammogram and ultrasound. Again I could tell by the looks and fake smiles and attempts at "nice weather we're having" conversations that something was serious. I had a consultation with a surgeon who suggested that then and there I have a biopsy. I'll receive the results in two days. Again, just by listening to the people working on me I knew. "I'm so sorry." "You did everything you could." I feel like I am having an out-of-body experience. I am not the same person who left my home this morning for a routine annual checkup.

I called Colin from the hospital and he came immediately. I feel so far away, as though I am moving in a different world. We had family time when we told the boys and the dog. They all were uncharacteristically silent. Michael cried and said, "There is no cure." Kids study lots of biology these days. Mark was his usual quiet, reserved self.

I don't feel much like telling anyone else until after the biopsy results. I just want to stay in my house with my husband and sons and dog and cat. I feel like cleaning out drawers and closets.

Today we went to the doctor's office for the results of the biopsy. I found out that I do have cancer. It is Good Friday. In a strange way it is better to know than not know. My first reaction was relief, "Well, now I know." Then I burst into tears and said, "But I have two children." The doctor responded that I'd dance at their weddings. Colin is very teary. I was handed lots of literature about wigs and turbans. Wait a minute! I have

In Colin's Words

I was at my desk in my office when Mary Ellen called me and told me that something had turned up in her routine annual gynecological exam. She asked me to come down to the hospital breast center where she was being examined. The shock of that call and its message was total. Mary Ellen is everything in my life, and the thirty years we have spent sharing our dreams, our feelings, and our love have been the only true period of happiness I have known.

I tried to be as much there for her as I could and to take care of all her needs. I tried also to be her cheerleader in a pragmatic rather than in a Pollyanna way. I wanted to be someone to whom she could talk freely, to whom she could express any fear or panic, however irrational. She is the center of my life, and I wanted to do anything that could improve her chances or lift her spirits.

Especially at the beginning, it was not always easy. To become a successful cheerleader, I had to put myself in a position where I had some cheer to offer. Partly because I had lost my own mother to breast cancer when I was a teenager and partly because of some irrational horror of medical drugs and procedures, I had first to make peace with my own sense of panic and inadequacy before I could give her all the care and encouragement she needed and deserved.

As Mary Ellen and I made the first round of doctors and tests, the news seemed to get progressively worse. It became clear to me that Mary Ellen's cancer was serious and that she would need all the support I could give her to deal with all her treatments.

In those first days, while we were waiting for her treatments to begin, I became overwhelmed with my feelings of fear, anger, and panic. For a period of two to three days I found myself in a weeping jag. Anything or nothing would set me off and, although I think I hid it from our children, I couldn't hide it from Mary Ellen. Perhaps for myself I needed to hit bottom before being able to devote all my energies and love to Mary Ellen and her ordeal.

So we started our journey together through a year that, as the oncologist warned us, was going to be long and hard. I acquired a new respect for Mary Ellen's strength and endurance, and my love for her grew as we battled the common enemy together. I had heard that cancer makes everything different in a family, but no one told me that all the differences are not for the worse. ●

always hated wigs and weird looking head wraps. I have a full head of curly hair that I love. I am not ready to listen to any "bald" talk.

We went to the Botanical Garden for a walk. Why is the garden filled with so many statues of women baring their breasts? And they always have two! Colin said he wondered what ever happened to all the statues of generals on horseback.

It is Holy Saturday. I went to church to help decorate for Easter. I told Father and my friends. We all sat down and they laid hands on me and prayed. Well, now I have told someone.

I don't feel like eating.

I had a session with my therapist. I wept. He encouraged me to write down all the questions I want to ask the doctors. And, whatever they say, Colin and I should take our time deciding what to do. Maybe we could refuse any treatment, take our Social Security and move to Ireland, where our money will go further. We talked about using the opportunity of having cancer to finally have the life I really want. What do I really want?

I love my family. I love my friends, and I love my neighborhood. I love my garden. I love my pets. I love life and living.

I finally told Colin my biggest fear: the cancer has spread beyond my breast, there is no treatment, and I am going to die.

Today we went to see an oncologist. The waiting room was full of very sick people—I couldn't look at them. I know I am not that sick. The doctor was very calm and took lots of time. The cancer I have is a very aggressive type, so a very aggressive treatment is recommended. He suggests chemotherapy first, then surgery, then more chemotherapy, and then radiation followed by five years of medications. I asked him about reconstruction. He agreed with the surgeon that I should not have reconstruction right away. The tumor is against my chest wall and the doctors want to be able to see my chest wall after the mastectomy. More will be known after the surgery when they see what kinds of margins they get around the cancer. Apparently, the better the margins, the less chance of recurrence at the site. I asked if he agreed with the surgeon

*that I would dance at my sons' weddings. He said, "Well, I don't know."
I stopped breathing. Then he continued, "It depends... do you know
how to dance?"*

> *In a strange way, I hope that cancer does teach me to dance.*
> *The doctor has ordered lots of scans and tests.*

*Today I prayed, meditated, and read for a long time. I saw Mary and
had a session with her. I asked her to help me—to be a member of my
team. I firmly believe that healing and wholeness are in the future for
me. I will be treated for cancer by my medical team. I will be treated
medically and scientifically. In addition, I will see Mary weekly. I will
consult with a psychologist whom I refer to as my coach. I know I need
a team to get me through this. I need my doctors, my family, my friends,
treatments, meditation and prayer, and my team.*

Mary Ellen has just found out she has breast cancer. She was pretty
measured and calm in the face of this. She wants to utilize all she
knows about healing to help herself. Would I be willing to give her
regular *Trager* sessions throughout her treatment?

This request has a new twist. I've had some patients with breast
cancer. Usually, I see them for residual difficulty with shoulder movements after treatment is completed. Others I've seen for a session or
two of *Trager* to explore its benefits to them. Now, here's a request for
weekly sessions during the entire cancer treatment. I would have to
clear this with the oncologist. I'll have to be accommodating to someone who is going to feel very sick at times. Our relationship would last
a whole year. Am I up to it?

I think the *Trager* Approach would potentially provide a calming
influence in a time of upheaval. It's very gentle, and that would be
important. Even though there will be unique situations to manage, I feel
very open to what could be a time of growth and challenge. And as my
mind busily evaluates the request, I really can't think of any reason not
to assist Mary Ellen in this way. If I could be of some help to her,
nothing would please me more.

During the *Trager* session today, during the part when I was
supporting her upper back and shoulders with my hands,
Mary Ellen told me she was aware of all the people praying for her
and supporting her.

*T*oday I feel fear again. An ocean wave of fear is washing over me. Fear is so debilitating. I try to embrace the fear. And I talk about the fear. I do not have to BE fear. Fear is partly overcome by knowledge. I am going through with the tests.

It is Sunday, and I went to church. I feel very odd and out of it. I feel like I have crossed a great, wide river, and I look back and see all my family and friends on the other side. Somehow I know I can never go back across and have it be the same. They are on the side without cancer, and I am on the other side, and I can never go back. I feel millions of miles away from everyone. My prayer is very simple, "Lord I believe, help my unbelief." The reading was about Thomas the doubter. That was very reassuring.

I just want to turn the clock back to the day before I was diagnosed with cancer.

Colin and I went for a walk in Tower Grove Park. Then we sat on a bench, and I just put my head in his lap, and he rubbed my back. The breeze was so refreshing and cool, and the grass and flowers are so lush. All the people walking through the park look so normal—do they ever think about dying?

A thought is just that—a thought. I am not my thoughts.

3 a.m. I am overwhelmed by terror and fear that I have cancer through-out my entire body. I have never known terror like this. I am sitting on the toilet, feeling terror. I have a bone scan today. I got some meds to help with my claustrophobic feelings in the scanner. The claustrophobic panics that first arose when I was trapped in the overturned car in the accident show up every now and then.

My sister picked me up for tests, and I told her how I was feeling. Before she arrived, I called or e-mailed some of my friends to ask for their prayers. I tried to stay with my breathing as much as possible. When we got to the hospital I asked to go to the room where the scanner was so I could look at it with my sister. Then they injected me with some kind of "glow in the dark" liquid. The room I was in reminded me of the old bomb *shelters, because of the little yellow nuclear windmills on all the signs. I told everyone I met who was wearing a white coat that I felt claustrophobic in those scanners! They were so great to me. With their help, God's help, the prayers of my friends and family, my sister, and my pills, I made it!*

Middle of the night. A terror night. I am afraid to look at my pathology report. I am afraid to go to a support group meeting at the hospital, because someone is there to help me read my pathology report and there may be stuff in there no one has told me. What grade is the cancer? What stage? How long do I have? What this? What that? Who wants to know?

Went swimming today. I love the feel of my body in water. I love to move in water. I am so free and borderless and edgeless and light. I can fly.

I worked up all my courage, called the surgeon's office, and his wonderful, fabulous nurse told me that my bone scan is clear.

I went to the support group meeting at the hospital last night. The speaker was a pathologist. I brought my pathology report sealed and unopened. The speaker reported much too much scary information for me to take in just now. I learned that each cancer is individual. Thus, what happens to one person does not necessarily happen to the next. I won't know the entire picture until the lymph nodes are checked postmastectomy. I noticed how the people with the tiniest lumpectomies and biopsies asked the most questions. I just wanted to scream and run out of the door. This was not a good idea to come here. Way too much scary doctor talk.

Last night I had my first good night's sleep. I think that every little bit of taking charge of my cancer helps me. Why did I write MY cancer? I don't want it.

Today, Mary Ellen said the results of the bone scan are negative for cancer. She still must have a CT scan. She spent some time describing the experience of wondering if every little twinge from the body is more cancer. I asked Mary Ellen if she had asked the oncologist about receiving *Trager* sessions during treatment. At this she brightened. He appeared very interested in what *Trager* was and expressed no alarm or reservation. "That would be just fine with me," she told me he said.

During the *Trager* session today, Mary Ellen told me "you have a healing ministry." She expressed appreciation for being able to say what she needs during our session, of being heard and then responded to, specific to that need. She remarked on the difference in touch between *Trager* and a mammography exam.

My oncologist told me that I would have a very rough year. I know I need helpers, I need my team, and I need to take care of my body through this. Oh God, help me.

I have the most wonderful husband any woman could ever have. Colin means more to me than words could ever express. He is the love of my life, the smile in my eyes. He knows me through and through, and he loves me. He is finding all of this so hard but, in spite of that, he is doing all he can for me. I see the tears in his eyes. My sons are the sun and moon to me. I cannot imagine life without them. My brothers and sisters are the best there could be. Each one has expressed such love and concern. I love them. Catherine is a wonderful sister to me. She told me that I am the first thing she thinks of when she wakes up and that she offers her day for me.

Peg is my dear friend and the sharer of my heart talk.

I love the Napersteck tapes. When I listen to the chemotherapy tape, I assume a relaxed posture, breathe deeply, and imagine myself at my favorite beach in Michigan. I am surrounded by all who have ever loved me. In front of me is a fountain of bright liquid light, and my friends and loved ones let me know that it is time for me to take the healing liquid into my body. It is time for me to be well, to share my gifts, to love and appreciate who I truly am. These are the friends and loved ones who have loved and supported me all along. They want me to love and appreciate myself better and to take the time to be well. They let me know that they are always there for me, and that all I have to do is call upon them whenever I need them. This is so reassuring. I weep each time I listen.

I wake up a lot at night. The tapes help. Am I going to die?

Today I am afraid of all the side effects of chemo. I asked my husband to sit with me and read through some of the "gazillion" pamphlets we have been given. There is way too much information for one person. I don't want to read any of them. They are way too scary. So, I read a bit and then asked him to read the rest and let me know if there was anything I really needed to know just to get through the next half day.

This is wig week. I asked Fran to go with me.

    I've joined a support group at the Wellness Community. My oncologist told me about it. The group is made up of people who have been, or are presently going, through cancer treatment. I am joining the same group that a neighbor of mine belonged to who recently died. She had had cancer for a long time, and I have watched her slowly die. Do you graduate from the group by dying? Some of the members look so sick to me. But they are wonderful and supportive of one another, and I do know that here is a group who really understands where I am. They tell it to me like it is. For example, definition of chemotherapy: you lose your hair, feel like shit, look terrible.

SECOND OPINION DAY. *Before going to the MD, I had a session with Mary. I stayed in the present, experiencing the warmth of the air, the coolness of Mary's hands, the weight of my arms and legs. I feel so reassured when she lifts my shoulders. It reminds me of those who love me and are praying for me. I can feel them lift me and carry me along. I really need this right now.*

    I went to the second opinion doctor. It was awful, and I knew by the look on her face—more than anything—that I have a serious cancer. I wanted to know if she would suggest any course of treatment other than what the first doctor had suggested. Answer: "No."

    What would be different if I chose her over the other doctor? Answer: "The parking would be easier." Is this treatable? Answer: "Yes." Is this curable? Answer: "Yes."

    Then—without taking a breath—she added that I have a 60% chance of surviving more than five years. Who asked her? Then she went on about what stage the cancer is and how compromised my breast is, on and on—who asked her?

    I did not ask, but she had to say it—that 60%.

    Then she showed me the chemotherapy treatment room. I hated it. It looked like a bunch of electric chairs all lined up. What is with gray recliners? Do all docs go to the same ugly furniture store?

Colin said he is worried about me, because I'm being too good. It is OK to be down. You never know with the cancer gods though. There is something about appeasing those guys that I have to figure out.

Colin is so good for me. I am just afraid that all of this will be too much for him.

It is so hard for me to keep telling people that I have cancer. I feel like they look at me as though I said I AM cancer. I want to turn back the clock and be the way I was before the diagnosis. I feel so far away from everyone. Does anyone out there know what this is like?

The two oncologists I have met have very different approaches in talking to me. The second opinion doctor brought statistics, categories, stages, chances of survival. In about ten to fifteen minutes, she gave us the picture. The other doctor seemed in no hurry to categorize or give me the statistics. He had no clear and definitive answers. He asked me if I knew how to dance! (I am learning it is time to sing my own song and dance.) He came to the meeting with something I can only describe as humility, realizing he did not know me and what I brought to the table. He spent a long time—in excess of an hour—getting to know me. He spent time trying to understand the belief system I brought, and I wanted to know his as well. What kind of confidence do we both have in each other and in ourselves? He understood how crucial the support of my husband was at this time and included us both in all conversations.

If I am watching TV, and there is a doctor or hospital show, I turn it off. I cannot read the obituaries in the paper anymore.

The CT scan was negative! Mary Ellen has also been for a second opinion, which yielded the same information regarding the treatment protocol. However, the doctor was too straightforward, unfeeling even. So, Mary Ellen will stay with the first oncologist she saw and the regimen he suggested.

I want more than ever, to be a contrast...no...an antidote, to the second opinion doctor. I sat in my chair facing Mary Ellen, who was propped cross-legged on my massage table, wiping tears away. Does Mary Ellen feel understood by me? I just listened, waiting until we were both ready to settle down and begin the session.

Mary Ellen was more teary today than usual. "This is so scary. I don't know if I can do it." She told me she's feeling overwhelmed. I asked Mary Ellen to focus on one thing at a time. This room, this experience. I felt my own anxiety rise as she hugged the pillow and rocked forward and back, still crying. Gently, I insisted. This room. This experience. This table. The color of the carpet. The amount of sunlight from the window. I talked through much of the hands-on work to keep her present. This feeling. This delightful movement. Slowly the tension in the air began to dissipate. We just practiced being here right now.

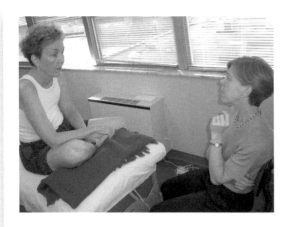

Between some quiet, deep breaths Mary Ellen whispered: "I'm not sure where my arm begins and the pillow ends."

I'm so grateful for these moments. It never ceases to amaze me how beautifully Mary Ellen enters into the dance with me, allowing the gentle movements to happen.

After easing ourselves out of the office, Mary Ellen borrowed my copy of *Imagery in Healing* by Jeanne Achterberg.

*H*ad a session with Mary. She suggested we each keep a journal and then put them together when the treatment is over. I like the idea because I know she thinks there is a beginning, middle, and end to this whole thing. She thinks I'll live through it! I'll lean on her faith for now.

I'm reading Imagery in Healing, *given me by Mary. The mind is powerful in the healing process. The use of imagery can cause changes in the body. I can play a role in helping my body heal in addition to taking the treatments and medicines, even enhancing the effectiveness of these treatments.*

I told my therapist about the second opinion doctor. He told me that stats are for doctors. Some docs like to sound authoritative, need to sound authoritative. They are supposed to know all that stuff. However, diseases don't read textbooks. Each cancer is unique, just as each patient is unique. I have chosen doctors I trust. I have my family, my friends, my prayer team, my neighbors, my parish team, my therapist/coach, Mary for bodywork. I will meditate and pray and live in the present.

I have been given an opportunity in my life to go on a retreat. During this time I am going on a spiritual journey. I am going to explore my life, my world, and my universe. I am going to ask questions and listen for answers. I am going to let the real Mary Ellen come to life. I am going to explore just what I want the second half of my life to be. What do I want to do? I embrace this time that is given to me.

I asked the doc for a Port-A-Cath®. Mom had one. I don't like the way they dig around my arms looking for veins.

My uncle has invited me to go to Lourdes with him. What a wonderful gift. I just cannot be away from Colin and the boys right now. I need to stay home.

I remember when we decided to adopt. I did not want to be associated with other people who could not have children. I did not want to admit that we had failed. I feel a little like that now. I belong to a support group for cancer patients. I have cancer. I have met and gotten to know other people who have cancer. Somehow, and I am not sure how, I have to admit something about myself. I move in a world I have not known before. It is difficult to accept this. I don't want this cancer. I don't want to go to a group. I don't belong there.

Hooray for life, hooray for love, hooray for family, hooray for husbands, hooray for children, hooray for friends, hooray for cats and dogs, hooray for butterflies and flowers, hooray for gardens. I love my life.

Today is Mother's Day and what a happy and privileged mother I am. I adore my boys, and I know how hard all of this is for them. I try to talk to them about it, but they are at an age where it is difficult.

I got my hair cut today. If it is going to fall out, I might just as well get used to it in stages. My sister came with me and gave me the haircut as a gift. I've been bald before. When I entered the convent, I did not know that hair cropping was part of receiving the habit. I felt so humiliated. I didn't recognize my face in the mirror. In winter, it was so cold.

In Michael's Words

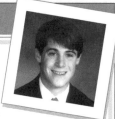

It was on a Wednesday after school, when I was a freshman in high school, that we found out that my mom had cancer. I knew that something was wrong hours before I even spoke with either of my parents that day. I carpooled with a friend that year—except on Wednesday afternoons when I had trumpet lessons at 3:30 and wind ensemble at 4:00. My mother would always be waiting to pick me up directly from school and hustle me over to the music school. Well, that Wednesday I waited outside for her for almost an entire hour. This was quite uncharacteristic of my mother. Often, if a conflict in her schedule arose, my mom would send word to me during school to find an alternate means of transportation. There was no message waiting for me. I called my mom at home, at her office in Kirkwood, and also at her office in Clayton; none of her coworkers had heard from her. I called my dad at work—he was not there either! It was about at this point that I suspected something certainly wasn't right. I managed to get a ride to the music school from someone at the high school; for some reason I had a sense of foreboding. The ride was eerily silent. After I explained to my private teacher why I didn't show and finished rehearsal with the ensemble, I again called my house in hopes of locating my mom. I was all set to give her a piece of my mind. There still was no answer. I set out to walk home. It wasn't a far walk, and I had done it many times before, but for some reason that day, I was very angry. I was preparing to really let my mom have it about forgetting about me and not even having the decency to call or leave a message. Sometimes, when I worry, I resort to anger and take it out in all the wrong ways. I was angry with my mom for having made me worry so much! As I was exiting a park close to my house, an even stranger thing happened. I saw that, for some reason, my dad was driving near the park, almost waiting for me. I got into his car and immediately knew something was wrong. He had a look in his eyes that was fearful. Naturally, I started to explain all the injustices that I had had to go through that day in order to get where I needed to be because of my mother's no-show. Almost immediately after I got in the car, I asked, "So where is Mom anyway, what's the deal?" To this he replied that she had been to the doctor that day and had some things she needed to discuss with the family. He would say no more. We arrived home minutes later and found my brother and my mom waiting for us in the living room.

"Daddy and Lou, have a seat. There is something I want to share with the family."

I sat next to her on the couch; my brother sat on the opposite couch, and my dad in his chair.

"I went to the doctor today to have my annual mammogram. During the screening, they discovered a lump in my breast. Nothing is certain at the present, but I had a biopsy and results should be known in a couple of days. There is almost no doubt, though, that it is a cancerous tumor."

I felt as if I had just received a blow to my face. This could not be happening, my mother did not just say that. Cancer? I knew about cancer; we had just finished learning about it in biology. *There is no cure for cancer. Its ultimate outcome is death.* These were some of the thoughts that ran through my head as I began to process this information. Immediately, and for a long time, I cried. My mom asked my brother to come over to the couch, and there she hugged us for what seemed like an eternity, while I truly began to despair. My dad joined us and, as a family, we sat there and hugged and were silent. I knew, concretely, that that afternoon marked an enormous transformation in my life, and to this day I have not been the same.

I cannot express in words the violent, turbulent, and brutal emotions that I experienced that afternoon. Indeed, I cannot even attempt to do justice with the English language to describe the massive anguish I felt that day. For 15 peaceful years, I had never given thought to the reality that my mother's days on the earth might not last an eternity. That was completely and utterly inconceivable to me. The impact my mother's cancer had on me was crushing. Through my sophomore year and into my junior year, I struggled with coping with my mother's illness. Indeed, her breast cancer rocked the very foundations on which I live and have built my life. It was for me a life-changing experience. ●

I wonder how I will look this time. Lisa was wonderful. She reminded me that she had done my mom's hair when she was receiving treatment. She has other clients who have lost their hair, so she knows the drill. Her smile and encouragement mean more to me than any haircut.

Mary Ellen had her treatment schedule lined out for her and told me about that. The mastectomy won't be until August or September. She had just come from having her hair cut shorter. It was Mary Ellen's idea to go a little shorter in preparation for the hair loss, but her sister came along and paid for the haircut. She got teary telling me this story.

Mary Ellen remarked on how she is guarding and feels protective of her left chest area. She said one of the reasons she likes coming here for sessions is that touch of her left side is reassurance and affirmation that she is OK, despite the breast cancer diagnosis.

Taking the box of *Wisdom Cards* from my desk, I opened the box and fanned the cards out on the massage table where Mary Ellen was sitting. She chose one and read it:

"I listen with love to my body's messages. My body, like everything else in life, is a mirror of my inner thoughts and beliefs. Every cell responds to every single thought I think and every word I speak."

I chose one, too.

"It is only a thought, and a thought can be changed. The thoughts I choose to think and believe right now are creating my future. These thoughts form my experiences tomorrow, next week, and next year."

We compared our messages for the day, and let the meaning sink in. This small ritual has become a pleasing way to transition from conversation to the quieter attitude needed for the *Trager* work.

I began, and we began. Whether with her head or her foot, I wanted my hands to convey what they know to be soft and easy in the movements. Yes, the left shoulder and arm, ribs and belly, forearm and hand, all get to move. They get to be held individually and together. Movement of one part, fanning out to the others. But this happens throughout the whole body, not just the left side. Mary Ellen said, "For a moment, I didn't remember I had cancer."

*W**ent to try on wigs. Everyone was acting so happy—like what a great treat that you can try on all these cute wigs and turbans. I thought they all looked horrible. I did not know that they do not make many wigs for curlies. You have to buy a straight one and curl it yourself. Curlies never curl their own hair! They don't know how! I just held back the tears through the whole ordeal and got out of there as fast as I could.*

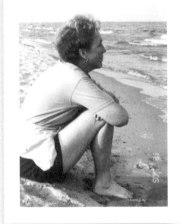

I am working on relaxation. (Did I write that?) I have a tape that is helping me get into a relaxed place using imagery. This weekend I plan to go to the office. I want to do normal things; I am feeling overwhelmed right now. Maybe if I try to pass for normal that will help.

When I listen to my imagery tapes, I am asked to relax, get into a comfortable position and listen. I go to my favorite Lake Michigan beach where it is safe and peaceful and beautiful. I make it as real as possible using all my senses. I am encircled by my loving friends, family, and well-wishers who see me surrounded by a healing light. This light illuminates any cancer cells in my body, so they can be taken care of by my body's own cancer-fighting mechanisms. Along with cancer, this light illumines any old hurts, resentments, and guilt that I hold on to from the past. It is time for me to forgive others and forgive myself. It is time to make space inside me for joy, gratitude, and peace.

Michael was in a recital today. I stayed completely out of any preparation, because I know I have to reduce stress. I learned that he can handle these situations, and it is really better for him that I stay out and let him make his own decisions. The same applies to Mark. He did not want to attend the baccalaureate Mass. I let him express his anger, and I stayed out of it. Let it go, let it go, let it go.

SPRING

Colin and I talked about retirement today. I hope to live long enough to retire with him. I can't bear the thought of dying and leaving him and my boys.

The Port-A-Cath® ordeal is over. "Very simple procedure, outpatient, home quickly after it is over." I guess I should have known something could happen when the last thing the doc said as she was marking my chest with her ballpoint pen was that, because I am so thin, they will have to use a different type of needle for the procedure.

I guess they used the fat needle after all, because my lung was punctured. So, I stayed overnight in the hospital hooked up to several machines measuring whatever they measure that then sets off alarms if the numbers are wrong. Next to me was a big, long tube just in case all hell broke loose, I guess. I could only imagine what they would do with that, since they did not go into detail. During the night I rang for the nurse, because I needed to be unhooked so that I could go to the bathroom. No one came, and I really had to go, so I unhooked myself. Alarms went off. I went to the bathroom fully expecting a squadron of scrubs to come running. I got back in bed, alarms still going. I could hook myself back up, but I did not know where the reset button was. I rang again. When the nurse finally came, she explained that the reason no one came in response to the alarms was that my room was too far away, and they could not hear anything. I stayed awake the rest of the night watching the numbers for myself. A "zillion" chest x-rays later, they told me that my lung had reinflated. My sister Catherine stayed for part of the night with me. I asked her to forgive me for those times when I was not a real sister to her. I told her I was sorry. I have needed to do this for a long time. She asked my forgiveness as well. We agreed that, from this night forward, we would start over and not bring up the past.

FIRST CHEMO. *I didn't sleep. I called my oncologist at 7 a.m., crying and shaking. I asked him if he was positive that this was the treatment I needed. Was he certain this would help me? I just don't know if I can do this. He told me that he understood how frightened I felt, because this was a rigorous course of treatment. Colin came with me, and I took my tapes. He sat at the foot of the recliner and massaged my feet. I didn't feel much like talking. I just focused on breathing, relaxing, doing imagery from my chemo tape. Afterward, my urine looked like red Kool-Aid.*

*My body knows that it has undergone something very different.
It feels like the underground rumblings before a volcanic eruption.
I am taking antinausea meds. I am very constipated.*

I received a card from a friend:

*"We are healed when we can grow from our suffering, when we can
reframe it as an act of grace that leads us back to who we truly are."*

Maybe the more I am who I truly am, the healthier I will be.

*I feel so shaky about going to a hospital and having surgery. They
punctured my lung. Who knows what else could happen? They are so
powerful. They are so understaffed. I am so scared.*

*Someone in my support group called cancer treatment "poison, slash,
and burn." In my case it is "poison, slash, poison, burn."*

*I lay in bed thinking that a part of my body is diseased. A part of
the body that I love is so diseased that, unless it is removed, I will die.
The nights are so long when I am so sick. Sometimes I wake Colin, and
he just holds me and we talk. Tonight I talked to Colin again about the
mastectomy. What will I be like? He repeated to me what he has said
so many times, that he loves me; he loves my eyes, my shoulders, my
breasts, and every part of me. If I have to have any part of me removed,
that doesn't change anything about the love.*

*Colin has joined a support group at the Wellness Community for family
members of cancer patients. I am so glad. This is difficult for him and
difficult to talk to me about it. I can see the pain in his eyes. Sometimes
I see tears in his eyes. I miss him so much when he goes to work or to
his support group.*

*How will I look after surgery? I find this difficult to imagine. My support
group listens. I have the name of a woman who sells prostheses. Can't
do that yet.*

*One of the steps in the 12-Step Program is asking forgiveness. I think
this is a step in any healing. Asking my sister's forgiveness, and having
her accept my apology, is a real gift to me and allows me to put down
burdens from the past and not carry them any further in my life.
Carrying forward old hurts and resentments from the past saps me of*

energy, when my energy is so low. Harboring old injuries and wanting someone to be blamed for what has happened to me makes me a victim. It also means that I am always on the outside, holding others at arm's length, while I wallow in the injustices done to me. I attach myself to my anger. I have a wonderful sister. I think that sometimes I got energy from stirring up old wounds from the past. I would excuse my need to change and move on. It is so much easier to blame someone. I did that, and it no longer works. Time to grow up. I don't think this is forgive and forget. I need to remember the experience and learn from it. We each forgave, and we each were forgiven. As I face the possibility of my own death, I see things much more clearly.

Into the valley of the shadow
the valley of the shadow
valley of the shadow
of the shadow
the shadow
shadow

©*Jan Newhouse, 2000*

SECOND CHEMO. *I took my tapes, a picture of my family, a rose from my rose tree, my soft pillow. Going down there this time felt worse than the first time. I felt very drugged and seasick all day. About 7 p.m. I vomited with such force that it was terrifying. Now I know how powerful the antinausea meds are. I have never experienced anything like this before. Now I know why they start you on antinausea drugs right away. I waited too long. Colin and Catherine sat with me.*

Peggy and Fran took turns sitting with me. I don't feel good about being alone.

Working with Mary is a godsend. Cancer treatment makes my body feel like it doesn't belong to me. I have pains I have never had and limitations I do not recognize. But Mary can take any movement I have, even the slightest, and make it seem that my whole body feels softer and better.

When I can't sleep I imagine myself on Mary's table and try to recreate that softness.

Today I went to the annual birthday party lunch. I have known each of these women most of my life, but today I felt so foreign. I remember just how I felt, year after year, sitting at these lunches. Today I felt like a stranger. They are all talking about their plans and projecting themselves into the future. What is my future? Do I have a future?

Fran brought dinner. I wept a lot with her. I can feel the anger that I have not let myself feel slowly coming to the surface. I have not let myself feel angry, because somewhere I feel that it is my anger that has caused the cancer. Deep down, I wonder if I have given myself cancer.

Spoke to Peg about my anger. She said to keep it close to me and know it is there ready to serve me well. Anger is energy, and I can surely use some of that right now.

Brought my feelings of anger up with my therapist. I talked to him about thinking that, because I have not come to terms with a lot of anger, I have given myself cancer. He said that even though there are some folks who talk like that, there really is no research to support it. More to the point for me is asking myself, "What do I do now? Where, when, and with whom am I my best? Do I want to continue in my job?"

It is early morning. Colin is not awake. I feel agitated. I say the rosary, clean out drawers. The anger thing is there. I am anticipating a chemo treatment.

My hair is falling out. I ran my fingers through my hair and was amazed at the handful that came out. I knew it would happen, but now I know it really does just fall out.

My white count is so low I am on injections. I burst into tears when they said I would learn to inject myself. One more thing. I have to come to the emergency room if I run a temperature of 100 degrees or more. I have to stay away from the public. I can eat only those fruits that I have peeled myself. No salad bars. I have no ability to fight infection. I am so tired.

I told Mary that my ribs hurt on my left side and that I am afraid that means the chemo is not working. She simply laid her hands on my ribs, shoulders, etc., in her Trager *way. Touching transmits many messages. Jesus healed by touch. The message from Mary was peace.*

From Mary I have learned that I can feel pain and sickness in parts of my body, but I can also ask if there is anywhere that I feel OK. I was lying in bed feeling so sick and asking myself if there was any move-

ment that I could do that felt good. Raising and lowering my little finger felt fine. So instead of distancing myself from my pain-filled and sick body, I asked what part of my body could I move to remind me of what "feeling good" felt like.

Mary Ellen wanted to know if I had found out how the chemotherapy drug is eliminated. I mentioned to her last time that, because I touch so much of her skin in a *Trager* session, it is important for me to know if the drug is excreted through the skin at all. I shudder to think of doing *Trager* while wearing latex gloves! But, happily, that won't be necessary. I spoke to the medical oncologist's nurse who referred to a drug book and said that both Cytoxan and Adriamycin are excreted in the urine, not the sweat. Mary Ellen reported that the Kool-Aid color urine she had been passing was now normal color, verifying my information.

I wondered about the feeling of being on chemotherapy. Would Mary Ellen remain comfortable on the massage table? Would a wave of nausea sweep through her and disrupt our process? What about all that gentle rocking, would she find it soothing or irritating? Her comment during the session again today was that she has so much of her that is healthy. The *Trager* work confirms all that healthy part of her. "Cancer schmancer," says her friend the nurse. I looked over to notice that her furrowed brow had become smooth.

Some of the *Trager* work was done while she lay on her side today, because prone just isn't comfortable. Sometimes movements happen in my hands that are surprisingly free. It happened today with Mary Ellen's shoulder blade. She noticed it, too. This place we reach, this mutual sensing of ease in her body, can't be forced. It just happens. It's a moment of deep connection. It's why I do the work.

Summer

J am convinced that women with hair, eyebrows, and eye-
lashes model all those cute hats and turbans in the brochures for
cancer patients. They are not bald from cancer treatment. That is
why the hats fit, and they look so great. On me the hats fall down over
my eyes. I really need to stuff the hats with tissue paper to make them
look like they fit the way they were intended to be worn—over a head
of hair. Well, after attempting that, I discovered that I look like a woman
with a lumpy, crinkly head. It reminded me of my children when they
would walk around in their Pampers, all paper crackly.

Why is it that:
In the bathroom down the hall from the room where I receive chemo
infusion, there is a sign over the toilet: "If you are receiving chemotherapy
please flush the toilet twice." Do they think that you can get cancer
from a toilet seat or toilet bowl? Or, better yet, maybe they think the
pipes will corrode. And they are made of iron!

Why is it that:
We always talk about battling cancer, being cancer survivors, the war
on cancer? Is it helpful to those of us who have cancer to regard it this
way? I don't think that my oncologist meant that I had an opportunity
to go to war for a year. It is more like staying completely focused on the
task at hand. I have decided to follow a treatment plan. I have my team
of helpers. I trust them. I want to stay focused. It is about focusing, not
about doing battle with cancer. It is about staying in the present
moment.

Why is it that:
So many cancer patients are given a year or so of treatment and then
told that five years free of cancer will indicate they are fine and need
no further treatment. Where did they come up with these numbers?

25

My doc says he has no idea. It was probably a bunch of guys who thought half of ten years sounded like a good number! Each patient is unique, with a unique body, life situation, and reactions. There are some ninety-year-olds learning a new language and some thirty-year-olds who feel life has passed them by.

Why is it that:
There are no beauticians at cancer centers. Hair, skin, nails—they are all part of the deal with cancer treatments.

Reading the warnings on my prescriptions, I find myself wondering if there is a medication prescribed that encourages you to operate heavy machinery while taking the medicine. Otherwise I wonder if, during the flu and cold season, all construction grinds to a halt and the national economy with it!

Today, Mary Ellen walked in with a vase of two red roses from her garden. I was just so touched by this gesture of giving in the midst of so much suffering.

Before we began, she was feeling a motion sickness in her stomach, so she requested that I not rock her head. I asked, "Would it be OK to just hold your head and neck, no rocking?" "Yes, that would be OK." So when I came to the head and neck area, I just held the weight with presence. Mary Ellen lay on her back for the hands-on work. After 40 minutes, the motion sickness was gone. And her feet! She was really struck by how good her feet felt today during that part of the *Trager* work. "It's so nice to have a part of me that feels so good."

That walk from the parking garage to the doctor's office is so-o-o-o-o long. Why don't they have benches along the way? I am so exhausted, and I have lost my sense of balance. I did mention the benches to a few people. But when you are able-bodied, you do not see long passage-ways as challenges. I often wonder why doctors' offices all look alike. Same old chairs along the walls, outdated magazines, cheery faced ladies asking to see your insurance card. I think I have waiting room phobia. What if all docs did not buy their waiting room furniture from the same gray, brown, and navy blue chair salesmen? How about recliners with soft blankets and pillows—and not that awful plastic? Has anyone ever thought of an office where you could wait in a hot tub, have a foot massage, or listen to relaxation tapes via headsets? How about an aquarium and a sandbox? And then there could be cups of tea and fresh flowers. When you are on chemo, you are just plain sick and exhausted. How about a room filled with all kinds of art supplies so patients could reframe their illnesses, express their hopes and fears, and play?

Traditional medicine assumes you are sick and treats you accordingly. The odd thing about breast cancer is that I felt fine until I began the treatment that was designed to make me sick in order to treat my disease. I wonder if it would be better not to tell us every single horrible remote possibility of side effects from chemotherapy. When you are set up to expect the worst, it often becomes self-fulfilling.

When I look in the mirror, I do not know who I am looking at.

Cancer treatment sends shock waves through my body. It is as if a voice in there is saying, "What are you doing? Do you have any idea how devastating this treatment is? And yet you keep going back for more." When I go to a session with Mary, I feel like I am bringing a body with me that is just screaming for some relief. When I get on the table, I realize how different this experience is from getting into a recliner for an infusion of chemo drugs. Here, I am receiving positive messages. Here, I am asked to stay in the present moment. Through touch and movement I remember what it was like to be well, to be free of pain. I also can spend time away from the fear that grips me. Mary is very quiet, peaceful, focused. She is a great listener. I do get the impression that she is not only listening for words, but that she also listens with her hands, and she communicates with muscles, bones, tissue—all that part of me that I don't want to think about just now. She is letting my body know that it can feel better, calmer, and more peaceful. Sometimes, through a movement, a memory comes to me, from where I do not know. Sometimes I start to cry, and I do not know why. When I tell Mary about this she says that is fine, whatever is there is fine.

In order to comfort me, some people tell me that God gives us only what we can handle. God knew that I could handle this disease. I really do not think there is a God who operates that way. I think that life has enough problems and complications without having to think that God has designed one specifically for me. This is part of what it means to be human. Rather than asking, "Why me?" I think the question is "Why not me?"

M ary Ellen arrived wearing a long, blond wig and sunglasses. "Do you think my wig maker captured me pretty well?" Then, when inside the room, there were tears about the upcoming chemotherapy treatment. What could she do to help calm herself?

Together we came up with a lot of ideas including affirmations; looking at a picture of her boys; remembering *Trager* sessions; visualizing white light/yellow light over the breast; visualizing all the people who love her, holding their light out to her; Colin rubbing her feet. At the end of the *Trager* session, Mary Ellen suggested I hire a van to come pick up people and the massage table as one piece and take them home. She was "so-o-o-o comfortable." Just wanted to stay put.

At the beginning of this session, Mary Ellen had been beside herself with worry about how to make it through yet another chemotherapy treatment, and, at the end of ninety minutes, she had attained a deep state of comfort, imagining how she might magically transport herself back home, still lying on the massage table. I asked her to simply notice the series of movements in her legs, arms, and back as the *Trager* session proceeded. Simply that: one series of moves after another. Pauses, and more movement felt, until ninety minutes had passed and the session was over.

I t is just before my third chemo and I feel better. I don't have diarrhea. My appetite is better. I'll know better how to manage side effects this time. I will take the antinausea meds right away.

From Mary I have learned what a beautiful, healthy body I have; its movements are musical and magical. The way my body moves in space is a wonder to me. I have learned that I can use imagery in order to help myself relax, center, breathe and heal. This is particularly helpful at night, when my imagination tends to work overtime reviewing the past. That is when I am most able to lie quietly and remember what my body felt like during the session. I begin with my legs, my strong flexible legs that have helped me all my life. I remember the lifting of my shoulders and the thought I associate with that—all my praying friends and loving family and friends holding me and supporting me. I feel the lifting of my head and neck and realize that I am not alone in holding my head high and facing this disease. I remember the many, many deep breaths associated with a Trager *session, and I focus on the air filling my lungs and moving through my body making it lighter. I use the exhale to rid myself of stress and toxins. I remember what it feels like to sink into the comfort of my body and to rest there. I know how fluid the movements of my body are, how graceful, how grace-filled and how beautiful. Mary is teaching me to slow down, to stay in the present, to delight in all my blessings. I am also taking better care of my body as a result. I have stressed my body in the past, and it has broken down. Now is the time to learn to love my body, to care for it, to cherish it, to delight in it, to thank God for it. I think I need to spend more time dancing!*

THRIVING TACTICS

1/2 day at a time
stay in the present moment
breathe
stay close to my dog and my cat
never go to a treatment alone
look at the New Yorker *cartoon collection frequently*
watch A Makeover Story
watch A Baby Story
frequent foot massages
look at old photographs
have docs I love and trust
have my team I love and can rely on
do crossword puzzles
lots of fun hats
lots of reflection time
laughter
lots of hugs

The massage from a friend, e-mailing everyone, meds, meditation and prayer. I am surrounded by love and prayer. My team is with me.

Yesterday I was very sick. I have just enough energy to get from my bed to the bathroom and back.

I have a metallic taste in my mouth all the time. It feels like I am sucking on a penny or a nickel. I always laughed at the kids for putting ketchup on everything. Now I do! All my taste is gone, except for the metal. I never realized how much I would miss the taste of a Coke. So I put lots of salad dressing on everything, hoping to taste it. Yesterday it was scrambled eggs. Or I put ketchup on everything, thinking I will taste that. Maybe I am hoping to eat with my eyes.

TOOLS FOR CHEMO TREATMENTS
My husband
Down pillow
Tapes and CDs
Photographs

The infusion nurses at the office are so understanding. I know that they see people like me every day, and they must wonder which of us will make it.

Is it possible that I am living and dying at the same time? Are we all doing that and we just don't realize it?

I sat in my living room and looked around it marveling at all that I have. I am so blessed that, if I never acquire another possession, I still have so much. I have loving friends who bless me every day with their friend-ship. I have a loving husband whose devotion is indescribable in its comfort and support. I have two loving sons whose love for me is so apparent and whom I love more than words can say. I have a loving family who cares for me. My sister Rita is arriving tonight to stay with me while Mark and Colin go to the University of Iowa for freshman orientation. Catherine comes over every day, and her presence is a loving and caring comfort for me that I could not do without. My brother and his family have lovingly prepared my bedroom, where I spend a lot of time. My friends and neighbors have organized and are delivering dinners to our house. Cancer has taught me to look around and see my blessings, and there are "zillions" of them.

On the in breath—present moment. On the out breath—wonderful moment.

Mary has taught me that so much pain relief comes from softening and lightening the muscles in the area of the pain. I have learned that softening and lightening toward others and myself is all part of the healing, especially the healing of the past.

When I look in the mirror, I do not recognize myself—no hair, swollen face, my eyes have changed. I feel like I am living inside a stranger's body.

What is this cancer teaching me? What changes do I need to make in my life? There are lessons for me here. One is about anger. I have cells growing out of control in my body, growing chaotically and directionless. What is the lesson here?

Wigs: hot, uncomfortable, not curly. The best use of a wig is filling out a hat.

Just came from my group. Lots of sick people right now, sick and discouraged. I feel very down. Maybe this group is not the best place for me right now.

I am learning to ask my body, "Where is the tension and how do I hold it? What does this tension feel like? What is free, light and easy? What does free, light, and easy feel like?"

It's Monday and Mary Ellen was looking forward to leaving for camp Miniwanca later today. But, oh, she was feeling fatigued, very, very fatigued—feeling not herself because she is someone "with pep and energy." The tears flowed. I'm sure I have no idea what this must be like for her.

I took a wait-and-see attitude about the value of a *Trager* session today. I offered the messages of ease, openness, and softness with my hands through the movements of the body. Checking in with Mary Ellen, I found that she did feel some of these comforts, but the feeling of fatigue was undercurrent.

This evening, I had a voice mail message from Mary Ellen. She had gone to the doctor and discovered her white blood cell count was very low, so she received additional Neupogen shots. Now she will have to wait until her white blood cell count increases before leaving town.

In Colin's Words

Our lives changed a lot once Mary Ellen's treatment began. She was scheduled to receive chemotherapy treatment in her oncologist's office four times, each separated by a three-week period, before undergoing the mastectomy operation. We had decided that I would take off work and accompany her to each chemotherapy treatment. I wanted to be part of the treatment process and felt that, by accompanying Mary Ellen, I would act as a second pair of ears to hear anything the oncologist or nurses said and also give her, by being there, a sense of being loved and supported. As I sat with her during chemotherapy, watching the poisons being dripped into her blood stream, I often found myself wanting to run away. I found that I needed to continually remind myself to place my attention on being there for her and not on the horror and distaste I felt for what was happening to her. As the tubes dripped slowly, she would lie quietly, sometimes listening to tapes and sometimes just meditating with her eyes closed. I would sometimes rub her feet, or read, or just try to concentrate on a general attitude of relaxed support.

Before going to each treatment, Mary Ellen and I would discuss questions and concerns we wanted the oncologist to address. Before the chemical treatment itself, we would have the opportunity to talk with the doctor after he gave Mary Ellen a physical examination. We were unusually fortunate to have a doctor who was never in a hurry and gave us all the time we wanted and needed. His attitude was positive and upbeat. He answered our questions and explained anything we wanted to know. I felt that my presence was especially valuable because, when Mary Ellen and I talked about the conversations later, we each heard different things and could reconstruct our memories with two pairs of ears.

Of course, most of our time was spent in the periods between chemotherapy treatments. I would go off to my work each day and perhaps talk to Mary Ellen once or twice. When I came home, I would expect to find her resting, sometimes with Catherine, her sister, sitting with her. Sometimes a friend or neighbor brought us a prepared meal, and sometimes I fixed something that I would try to make palatable to Mary Ellen and also to the boys and me. There was a rhythm to the periods between the treatments. In the first three or four days after a treatment, she had almost no appetite and often suffered from nausea. She also was fatigued in that period and for a great deal of the rest of the time.

After the initial four-day period, we began to worry about the effect of the chemicals on her immune system. Her white blood cell count went down, and I had to be constantly ready to rush her to the hospital emergency room if she showed any signs of inflammation or infection. As the second week drew to a close, the corrosive effects of the chemicals would slowly begin to wear off, and the final week would see Mary Ellen's spirits rise until the prospect of the next treatment drew close with its accompanying gloom.

My stress through all this didn't come mainly from having to prop up Mary Ellen's spirits. She constantly amazed me by the positive attitude she maintained, even when she was fatigued and frightened. What tugged me down was the fear I had for her survival and the plain fact that none of us, doctor included, knew at the time whether the treatment was going to be effective. Mary Ellen and I had a mantra we shared from the first days we knew each other: "We are going to make it!" and this time I really didn't know if it was true.

I found one source of support at this time that helped me immeasurably. At about the time Mary Ellen began treatment, I started to attend a support group for cancer caregivers and family members at the Wellness Community. The Wellness Community exists in a number of cities around the country. It provides cancer patients and their spouses and other family members with professionally led support groups and other services. It is privately funded, and all its services are free. I started going every Wednesday evening when I could. There was a group leader, Inge, who had twice been treated for cancer herself, and had come to the United States from Austria shortly before the Second World War. I found her style and methods personally helpful to me. In a very nondirective way, she encouraged us to share with each other our panic moments and our hopeful times, our exhaustion, our fears, and our feelings of stress. Each of the members of the group had a spouse, parent, child, or someone close to them being treated for various kinds of cancer. In age, background, and temperament we formed a very varied group but, because we all shared the same fear and stress, I found it was a place where I felt I could be open. I grew to trust the members and to become involved in their feelings and their stories and their lives. It meant a great deal to me to have one place where I didn't need to pretend and didn't need to put up a "front." Cancer and our love for its victims bound us together and formed us into a unique community. ●

SUMMER

*T*oo sick to leave for Michigan. Had blood count done, and I'm back on the shots. The car is all packed, and I just cannot get out of bed and get in the car. I'll try again tomorrow. Colin is being so patient.

Too sick again today. More shots. Maybe we can leave tomorrow.

About noon I made it into the car! I am taking filled syringes with me, so that I can inject myself for the next few days.

We arrived at Miniwanca for family camp. I've been so warmly welcomed by my friends. I did not realize how big this place is until I could not walk from my room to the dining hall. I made it down to the sandy beach, but I cannot get as far as the water. I sat for a long time on the beach, so grateful that I am here, so grateful to be in this place. I saw the sunset, and that is enough for me right now.

About midnight I lay on the beach looking at the sky. There was no moon. Because I am away from any ground light, I truly experience the bowl of the firmament. When I start trying to imagine the depth of the universe and the millions of light years represented there, I have to close my eyes because it is so overwhelming. My body knows where it came from and, each time I return to nature, I am returning home. I know I came from the earth, and I happily acknowledge my mother, earth. The light, the breeze, the colors, the silence, the stillness, the wonder— it is all inside me. And it all wants to be well.

FOURTH CHEMO. Today is my fourth and last chemo of the first round. I'll have a session with Mary before I go. I want to relax into the body I have now, with all the effects of treatment I am experiencing. I go to feel better in spite of them. What is this pain teaching me?

I have sand from my Michigan trip that I take with me. When I run my hands through it, I can see and feel myself on the beach in my space, and I can relax.

Here was Mary Ellen wearing her camp logo shorts and shirt, freshly back from camp! Her smile was beautiful. Her eyes lit up. Despite not being able to be as active as she usually is at camp, Mary Ellen announced that she had a great time, as did her son. Today she brought a Ziplock bag of Lake Michigan sand with her and planned to run her fingers through it during her fourth chemotherapy treatment later today.

In no time, Mary Ellen was lying on the massage table, looking ready and settled in. She told me a little bit about the sensations of chemotherapy, such as nausea and diarrhea, an ache in her sacrum, a metallic taste on her tongue, and fatigue. She went on, "When I come for *Trager,* you don't treat me like I'm sick." Mary Ellen said she could feel the parts of her body that feel well. "It's the great thing about *Trager.*"

My chemos are over. I did it. We did it. My team and I did it. Surgery is scheduled for August 31. My red and white counts are low, and so I am on injections for both. I am extremely fatigued all the time. I don't feel up to going out of the house at all. The family reunion is planned for this weekend, and I don't think I can face it. It takes too much energy to pay attention.

I'm just not used to seeing a bald cancer patient in my waiting room! Mary Ellen had a bright scarf tied around her head today. But it came off before we began the *Trager* work. The bald head is a change for both of us. I held that head, rocked and cradled that head during our session, and it's changed! No longer the hair that helped my hands slide, that insulated them from the intense warmth of a head. Now, I can feel the oils of the scalp. And skin, everywhere my hands go, skin! I didn't expect this! I'm not even sure what I expected. Certainly the absence of hair, but this was a wholly new feeling landscape! The detailed shape of the head became more defined as I continued to playfully explore its weight. Inside me, there was a hair tousling movement of my hand that wanted to join in the mix, but alas, no hair to tousle! Amused by this, by the feedback loop between what I was sensing through my hands and the gentle expression of connection and softness that came from them, I smiled.

Mary Ellen often refers to her head in my hands as a bowling ball. This makes us both laugh! From the things Mary Ellen says, being bald is a real shift in the feel of things. It's cold without hair! Then, too, everything sounds differently when her head touches the pillow, or a sweatshirt comes over the head, or a hat is propped on top. For the past several weeks, Mary Ellen has been startled to see a sampling of her hair left on the pillowcase after the *Trager* session.

I am preparing for surgery using more imagery tapes. They are a wonderful help to me. In the tape I am encouraged to picture an operating room in which there are doctors and nurses preparing for surgery. Then a patient is brought in, and I know that I am that patient. I am being wheeled into the operating room by all who have ever loved me, and they stand all around me wishing me well and pleased that I am taking this step to be well. They stay with me throughout the surgery, smiling and nodding, kind and caring, keeping me safe. They move me out of the operating room and into recovery, where they stay with me. My body now knows what it needs to do to mend. I am comfortable and safe, protected by love and care. I can now get better.

Hold my anger close. Maybe my anger can be valuable to me in helping me get well. It may hold the energy I so desperately need and, right now, I am completely out of energy. I need this energy to move on. It may help me see clearly just what changes I have to make in my life. Anger is energy. I'll take that in any form it comes!

What is all this pain teaching me? I do want to learn to dance.

Louise has given me a great book on surgery preparation. I have sent my surgeon a letter. In it I asked him to speak positively to me during the surgery, telling me how well the procedure is going and that following the operation I will heal well, be hungry, and urinate easily. I want only positive statements about my condition to be talked about during the operation. I want to be told how well I am doing and how quickly and successfully and fully I will recuperate. I want no negative statements made about my case or me when I am under anesthesia. I trust my doctor. I will bring a copy of this request with me to the hospital and pin it to my gown when I dress for surgery so everyone knows my requests. I will also bring my music tape to listen to during the surgery.

M ary Ellen arrived with flowers, cut from the Heman Park cutting garden. I appreciated her bringing brightness into our meeting today. She genuinely loves to look at each flower and marvel at it—the deep color of this one, the architecture of that one.

There were some tears in anticipation of the mastectomy next Thursday. Mary Ellen reviewed how she had sent a letter to the surgeon asking him to say certain things to her during surgery, such as, "Everything is going just fine," and "You'll be able to urinate without any problems when you recover from the anesthetic." She has many friends who will be praying for her during the surgery, and she has a friend who is a nurse who will stay with her in the hospital.

By her tears and words, I was brought to the very moment of a surgery that will disfigure a body while, at the same time, will rescue a life. Mary Ellen's journey presents hard bargains. She gifts me with her ability to grieve her anticipated loss. I sensed her preparatory mood as she lay quietly and breathed deeply, as if she was already in the surgical suite.

Where does worry go when we become quiet? Would I be able to feel it in the body? Would the sluggish movements that tense muscles create reveal it? Or would playful, bouncy movements distract and allow us both to lose ourselves in the moment? There were some of each here. We moved from one experience to the other and back around again. Yet, a mind searching for ease will find it.

M *astectomy: disfigurement or reconfiguration on many levels, not just the surgery site. When I feel pain and sickness in one part of my body, can I find other places that feel well, strong, light, free? Cancer treatment needs open channels.*

I am preparing for surgery by thinking of everyone who has ever loved me. When I was a child I interpreted messages from my parents, teachers, family members, or friends as meaning—when they said they loved me— that they expected something from me. I read that expectation to mean good behavior, responsibility, good grades. So, in exchange for love, I had to figure out what they wanted, how to please them. As I grew older and heard someone say they liked me, I immediately thought of the expectations they must have of me, and I feared that I would not be able to live up to them. This is not true any more. I do not have to be a certain way in order to be lovable.

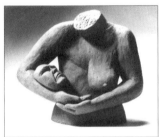

Nancy Fried.
Cradling
Her Sorrow.
Collection
of the artist.

S
U
M
M
E
R

Nancy brought me a pink fleece blanket today. When she was to have surgery, I suggested that she should imagine herself wrapped in a pink blanket. That blanket was my love and the love of everyone who cares for her, and who has ever cared for her. I asked her to close her eyes and imagine herself surrounded by all that love. Today she appeared at my door with a real pink blanket that she had made for me. Now it is my turn to have surgery, and I have a real pink blanket! Another comfort for me is that Mimi will spend the night of the surgery with me. That will help me feel safe.

I have a wonderful hat that I absolutely love—not so much for the hat, but because of the hatter who made it. When she saw me trying on hats with my bald head, she cut the price of the hat in half. We had a wonderful conversation, and we both went on our way having been blessed.

Mary Ellen was looking lively today, wearing a beautiful straw hat and carrying a mason jar full of flowers that she cut from Heman Park near the pool. I commented on her high energy level. Her younger son is leaving tomorrow for England, and she discovered yesterday that a dear friend of the family would be on the same flight out of St. Louis with her son! It was obvious how bowled over she was by this coincidence, so delighted, surprised beyond her imagining.

Our session today was quiet. Again, great care was taken with the right wrist and hand, because of the Port-A-Cath® in place on that side. Afterward, "I'm so comfortable, I don't want to move." She again asked for "the van to come pick me up and take me home." Ever the sense of humor.

Sitting up on the massage table, Mary Ellen, in a reflective tone, told me that she is very healthy, but that she just has a chronic illness. She has "L-M-N-O-P." And just like people with diabetes or emphysema, there are certain things that one must do if one has "L-M-N-O-P." One must manage stress, keep the immune system up, meditate, breathe, and visualize. She conveyed this scenario convincingly, complete with a brilliant attitude of confidence in her ability to do what is required.

*W*hen I was a child, our family would visit my elderly grandmother in Minnesota during the summer. My dad was a doctor, and part of the yearly trip always included a checkup for Grandma McShane. She would wait until the day before we were leaving and then ask my dad to check her heart, pulse, and blood pressure. She was always nervous during this ordeal and fingered her rosary throughout. To her great relief, she always got a good report and was told that she was fine and to continue doing whatever she was doing. I remember the look on her face—her smile—when the report was given, and the prayer book and rosary were laid aside until that evening.

One summer, a cousin was visiting grandma at the time we were there. She was studying nursing and asked my dad if she could check grandma's blood pressure and pulse. I remember being in the kitchen when my dad spoke to my cousin and told her that grandma was a very old woman, with a very old woman's heart. He told her that when she checked grandma's heart to tell her that her heart was working well and that whatever she was doing she should continue to do, because she was fine. So, they went through with the checkup and, again, grandma prayed throughout the ordeal. Then that wonderful smile and look of relief came over her face when she was told the results. Grandma lived well into her nineties.

Mark goes off to college today. I have written him a letter, which I will leave behind in his dorm room. We drove to Iowa and got his room all set up and then had a big family hug. It is great to feel like a mom and not like a cancer patient. I am relieved that both of my sons will be away from home during this surgery. I know they are worried, and we promised to call them immediately and keep them informed at all times. But it is time for them to go and time for me to focus on the task at hand.

Michael left last night for school in England. Father Luke was on the same flight, which was a wonderful surprise. Surgery is tomorrow. I am feeling positive; I have been using my tapes to prepare. I have been visualizing clear lymph nodes. I am feeling overwhelmingly loved and cared for and cherished by my family and friends. I have gotten so many cards, phone calls, and e-mails. Mimi will stay the night with me after the surgery, and I am feeling so calm as a result. We will really *know the extent of this cancer when all the test results are in after the surgery. God help me.*

I am not cancer. I have a chronic illness. I will learn to live with this.

It's Thursday. In mid afternoon I checked voice mail, and there was a message from Colin. He called to tell me Mary Ellen had come through the surgery "just fine" and thanked me for all my help.

Operation completed. It all went very smoothly. When I met my surgeon in the "green room," he had my letter in his pocket. He was happy to do as I requested in my letter. I spoke to the anesthesiologist as well, and she was fine about my requests. As soon as I got back to my room, about 1 p.m., I immediately went to the bathroom! I had a morphine pump and was able to keep myself very comfortable all afternoon and evening. In the evening a nurse came in and asked if I was in pain, and I said no. She asked me why I had not been requesting morphine from the pump. I said that I had been using it all afternoon and evening. After examining the pump, she found that it had not been working, and that I had given myself no morphine that entire day! The pump was finally fixed about 10 p.m. Mimi stayed the night, and that was the best comfort. By morning I had an excruciating headache, and I asked them to stop the morphine. Because of the headache and nausea, I stayed an extra day in the hospital and was able to go home feeling much better. Now my record reads "allergic to morphine."

This morning I asked Colin to stand with me in front of the mirror while I took my first look at the results of the surgery. I had no idea I would look like that.

In addition to the surgery site, I have small plastic jars that look like grenades at the end of drain tubes coming out of several places on my chest and side. These "grenades" have to be emptied periodically. I have to empty them and record the amount of fluid and the color. Their color wheel consists of blood, reddish-yellow, and yellowish-red. I call them Scotch and water, bourbon and water, cherry Kool-Aid, and lemonade.

In Colin's Words

A s the time came closer for her mastectomy, Mary Ellen became concerned about how her "disfigurement" would affect our relationship. It was not hard to be sincere in assuring her that all the important things that made her attractive to me—her intelligence, humor and vivacity, her eyes, her smile and, above all, her friendship—none of these would be changed by the loss of a breast. This did not mean that there would not be a pang, as there had been when she lost her hair (although that was only a temporary loss). Physically, her breasts were very special and to me particularly appealing but, as I told her, she could lose all her limbs without affecting the depth of my feeling for her.

The mastectomy operation itself came at a time when Mary Ellen and I were alone together. Mark had started his freshman year at the University of Iowa, and Michael had left for England to spend a semester abroad at my old school. That made it possible for me to concentrate totally on Mary Ellen and what was happening to her. To a considerable extent, this was only partially necessary, because she had thoroughly briefed her surgeon, her anesthesiologist, and the surgical team on what she wanted and needed! However, our previous hospital experience had shown us that the patient needs a watchful advocate. Mary Ellen, largely because of her preparations, came through the operation very well, in spite of the failure of the pain management system. After the first day, however, they wanted to release her from the hospital. Because she had reacted badly to morphine, when they finally administered it, and had a severe headache, she was dispirited, in some pain, as well as suffering a letdown from all the emotional energy she had put into making the operation successful. I found myself desperately tearing from one person to another in the hospital on a mission to find the one authority figure who would and could authorize a second hospital night for her. When, exhausted, I was finally successful, she became more peaceful and came home the next day in a more positive frame of mind. ●

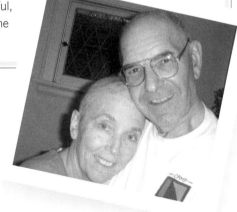

My anticipation was high today. I had talked to Mary Ellen since the surgery and heard the sound of her voice—accomplished, satisfied, relieved, mournful, searching. Today we would approach, together, the fresh scar, continuing to assimilate this latest alteration.

Upon her arrival, Mary Ellen's demeanor was subdued, the over-sized sweatshirt she wore was obviously borrowed. Once inside the privacy of my office she became more animated. First things first. Would I like to see the scar? Off came the sweatshirt to reveal a sleeve-less white T-shirt that was as much chamber as curtain. Two large silver safety pins pierced the fabric over the left side, hinting at the changed bodyscape beneath. With something close to pride, yet tinged with relief, Mary Ellen revealed the bandaged chest wall complete with exiting drain tubes. Collecting in fist-sized compartments at the end of the tubes was a small amount of amber red fluid. Then I noticed the culprits of the muffled clunk and clatter that had replaced the smooth, quiet presence of a breast. Gently untaping the uppermost boundary of the square bandage, Mary Ellen invited a peek at the stapled incision. I was relieved to see such a healthy looking incision, gently curving as it hugged the chest wall. I looked into Mary Ellen's eyes and saw that it was OK.

Bandage and T-shirt now back in place, Mary Ellen told me the story about how the morphine failed to find its way into her veins after surgery, unbeknownst to her. Hours later, when finally the equipment was fixed, the morphine actually proved to be too much for her. Morphine became a source of pain rather than salvation from it.

The *Trager* session was anticlimactic today, in a wonderful way. The surgical site was privileged—allowed to rest and have space and time to heal. As she lay on her back, I began with some movements of the legs. She asked that I really go slowly. She was talking a lot, processing the surgical event. After the leg work, I invited her into the feeling there, and she nodded a familiarity and noted how heavy and sunk into the table her legs had become. She was also comfortable lying on her right side, so we finished the *Trager* in that position. "That was really great," Mary Ellen told me afterwards. I observed her quieting and slowing down.

THE *TRAGER®* APPROACH

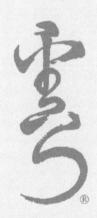

"Once an old woman came to Buddha and asked him how to meditate. He told her to remain aware of every movement of her hands as she drew the water from the well, knowing that if she did, she would soon find herself in that state of alert and spacious calm that is meditation."

SOGYAL RINPOCHE
THE TIBETAN BOOK OF THE LIVING AND DYING

Milton Trager M.D., the author of the *Trager* Approach, used touch, movement, and intention to communicate ease to the body and, ultimately, to the mind of the client. He called his work psychophysical integration.

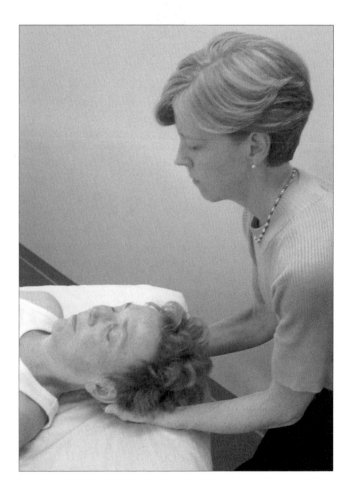

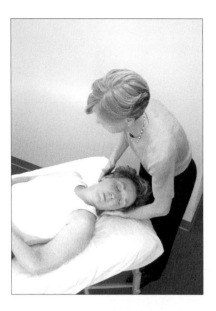

The *Trager* Approach is an educational process based on both passive and active movement of the receiver's body. The practitioner, through these gentle movements, communicates bodily ease to the client. The practitioner, through touch and movement, continuously searches for what can be softer, more fluid. The client opens to the series of movements as she is ready or able. Together the practitioner and client interact in a dance-like manner creating a feeling experience in the body. This experience often is one of deeper awareness, comfort, and ease.

The *Trager* Approach to movement education has been called variously neuromuscular re-education, skilled touch, and the Zen of somatic practices. The quality of touch is exceptionally gentle yet profoundly present. It is respectful and inquiring, never demanding or forceful. Often this style of touch is surprising or different to many people.

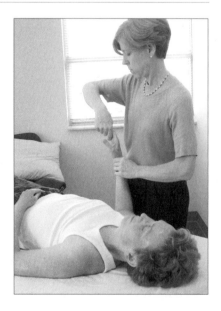

Introductory *Trager* sessions are usually choreo-graphed similarly so that, by the end of ninety min-utes, legs and arms, head and neck, belly and chest, shoulders and back, have all been touched and moved. In this way wholeness and completeness is communicated. The entire nervous system is spoken to. Integration of less known or less felt parts of the body can begin. This is usually accomplished by hav-ing the client lie on her back for part of the session and face down for part of the session. However, when these two positions do not provide the most comfort, alternative positions are used, such as lying on one side or sitting.

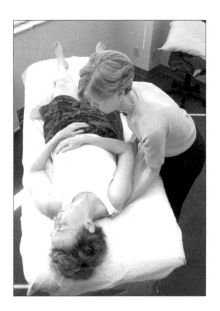

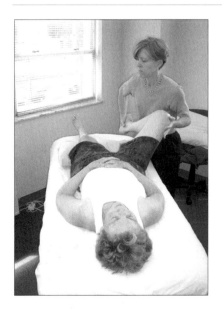

A *Trager* session is essentially a kinesthetic experi-ence, not a visual one, not an auditory one, not an intellectual one. So, customarily, the room that a practitioner and client share is quiet, except for the sound of a deep breath or sigh, or occasional requests or queries as the two continue to stay in touch. However, there are times when a client is unusually stressed, distracted, or emotionally upset that there is benefit to speaking one's experience as a practitioner. It opens another channel of input to an unfocused brain. It anchors more fully both the prac-titioner and the client in the present moment. The client gets to hear the musings of the practitioner while feeling the movements in her own body. Talking through a session like this deepens the client's sense of presence to the experience and is often helpful in diminishing her distracted, upset state of mind.

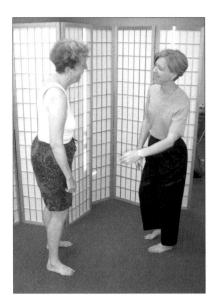

Mentastics® is the practice of the *Trager* Approach without the aid of the practitioner's hands. *Mentastics* is the contraction of the words *mental* and *gymnastics*. One learns how to bring awareness inward and feel the weight of different parts of the body, to use gentle swinging movements or effortless movements to get in touch with this weight. Giving oneself the experience of effortless movement over and over again creates changes in posture and movement. During *Mentastics* one brings awareness to the feeling state of the body and an openness to ease where ease was absent. In searching for how to be comfortable and open in the body, one enters into a creative process engaging the imagination, movement, and feelings. This is *Mentastics*.

"What can be easier, softer, lighter?" These are called the "Trager questions," used by Milton Trager to draw his students more deeply into their felt experience and to help them engage their creative mind—both the conscious and, especially, the unconscious mind. One uses the questions anytime, anywhere. They are invoked while doing *Mentastic* movements, as a reminder of intention. As the student feels movement, maybe walking or even just the movement of breathing, she can ask, "What could be easier?" The body will respond. The questions help in searching out where the effort is, providing the opportunity to let it go. The questions are meant to descend gently upon one's experience as a whole and to enlighten. There are no correct answers, only the response of the body to the questions. "What could be easier?" is also variously asked, " What could be lighter? How could this be? What would be more effortless? What is soft, and softer than that?" By entering into the query, one becomes open and expectant and very often feels a shift to a more comfortable way of being in the body, in the mind.

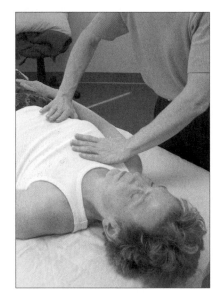

A final fundamental *Trager* principle is the notion of working "in Hook-up." This is the *Trager* language for the meditative state, for being in the moment, for being in the actual feeling experience of oneness with all. Call it deep gratitude. Call it speechless. Call it wonder. When teaching this attitude and state of bodymind, Milton Trager asked his students to remember what it is like to hold a newborn infant, and all the marvel and oneness of the moment that accompanies such an experience. Or he would ask them to remember when being captivated by a beautiful sunset or other moment in nature that seemed to make time stand still. This is the experience of Hook-up. It knows the present moment. It knows the truth of the connection of all beings. It knows the presence of a benevolence greater than ourselves. A *Trager* practitioner seeks to pause before beginning a session and bring herself into this meditative state. By doing so, the meditative state is imparted to the client. It is, in fact, the essence of the work.

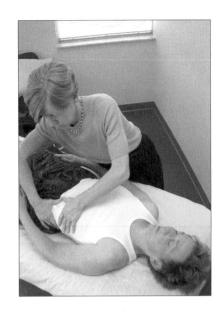

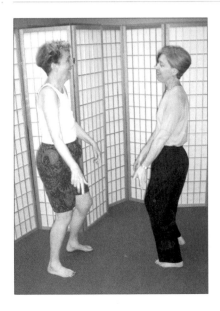

The *Trager* Approach uses movement as the ongoing focus of attention. Milton Trager taught awareness of "every moment of every movement." How the tissue moved, what areas of the body were moving, the rhythm that the body fell into, the timing or resonance of the movement—this is the information to gather into the container of awareness. This is the simple mandate, whether while creating movement in one's own body while practicing *Mentastics* or playfully exploring movement in the body of a client, one must just be there, noticing.

Autumn

Finbarr has a lump on his leg that is malignant. There is no treatment. I did not know that there is chemotherapy for dogs. So we will watch him, love him, and make him comfortable for whatever time he has left.

If I had known then what I know now, I do not know if I could have consented to treatment. It is the length of it. I'm so glad I didn't read every possible side effect. I just need to stick to my plan and stay focused.

If I ever write a book, it will be called **It's Not About the Disease.**

Why is it that:
The only people who want to talk about combat are the people who have never been in it. I have been asked: What is your prognosis? Do they think they got it all? What stage is your cancer? How many lymph nodes did they remove? Well, what do the doctors think? Has it spread?

One of the best parts about an appointment with Mary is that we laugh. I need that. I wonder if the Trager pantheon approves.

Had to have more coaching from my therapist about ignoring statistics. That numbers game haunts me at night. Who are the women in those studies? How were they selected? How does their situation resemble mine?

A woman called and left a message that she had visited me in the hospital as a representative of a recovery group. I do remember opening my eyes and seeing a strange woman at the foot of my bed. She wanted *to leave pamphlets and talk to me about doing exercises for my arm and prostheses and prosthetic bras. I remember feeling so overwhelmed that I burst into tears and told her I did not want to talk and not to leave me anything. Why would a perfect stranger think that, just hours after having surgery for a malignancy, I would like to talk? All I wanted to do was scream, "Get the hell out of here." I wanted her speech to be for someone else. Surely this must be a mistake. You can't be talking to me. You've got the wrong room.*

Asking friends to come for visits is wonderful. They are a big part of this recovery. My neighbors and parish friends are bringing dinners several times a week. I am so touched by all this. The boys are in their respective schools. Michael spent the first few days at his school in England in the infirmary with a sore throat and fever. Music lessons are set up.

I have an appointment with Mary on Monday, when we will begin nudging my arm. E-mailed the hospital commending Eileen, the night nurse. She was wonderful through a very long night. Some nurses really get it, and then the system overwhelms them, and they quit. She told me she is leaving soon.

My wardrobe now consists of an oversized T-shirt to which I pin my grenade collection and leave room for the drain tubes. Mary didn't wince or cringe when she saw the surgery site. We laughed about the grenades, and I asked lots of questions, because I feel more comfortable just now talking to Mary. She helped with frozen shoulder before. I do not want it again.

Surgeon's report: not good. There was lymph node involvement. Some lymph nodes were removed. The surgeon did not get the margins he had hoped for. The tumor was so close to my chest wall. The part I had dreaded is now fact. Now I know.

The docs tell me, "Exercise your left arm. Walk your fingers up the wall." Mary suggests that, when I do my arm exercises, I lie on my side. This is a lot easier than raising my arm from a standing position. Plus, we laugh.

M ary Ellen had a lot of tears about having to begin the second course of chemotherapy this Friday. I gave her a chance to express some of the anguish around this. She's just plain afraid. She described the additional struggle of living with discomfort as well as numbness in the area around the scar. This area is too sensitive even for the light touch of *Trager* right now, so I encourage Mary Ellen to bring kind attention to her healing surgical site by taking deep breaths or simply placing her hand there.

I have protected my left side so much that I have changed my posture. Mary has suggested that I open up my chest more. When I do that, maybe I am opening up my acceptance.

M ary Ellen told me about the first new round of chemotherapy—how she brings Play-doh, drawing material, and how she can visualize and feel the sand at the beach in Miniwanca. "I can feel it with my feet."

Today we have a discussion about participating with your mind in your healing. There is no guilt trip if you are not cured. Rather, there can be healing even if a person dies. "I don't know how, but I know this," says Mary Ellen. Difficult discussion. Mary Ellen got pretty quiet after that. Even though there had been tears earlier, Mary Ellen quieted, and, at the end, felt like she does "just before falling asleep."

A fter all this will I die anyway? Living or dying, is that the issue? Now is the time to embrace living, embrace dying, and make the necessary physical and spiritual changes. Whether I live or die, I must make room in my heart for joy, love, peace, and gratitude.

I am aware of how privileged I am to be able to afford this very expensive medical treatment, all because we have health insurance. Getting well is expensive, and good care is not available to everyone. The system needs a major overhaul.

AUTUMN

I am aware of how many times, in conversations with those in the healing professions, they will say that they would recommend something, but no insurance company will pay for it. It's as if there is a third party in the room during the consultation. This makes trusting difficult.

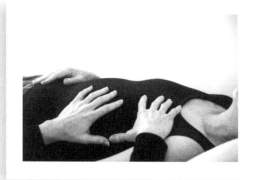

When I have a session with Mary, I feel more in charge of my cancer. I live in periods of terror and fear that cancer has taken over my whole body. I feel like a stranger in the land of my body. It is no longer familiar terrain. Each time I have chemo, I have no idea who or what I will be. My only roadmap is the pages of side effects that I am given to read and the medications to counter side effects.

I need to get back in the water.

Herceptin is my new ally in this plan. But, in order to take it in the usual chemo way at the doc's office, I have to get my first treatment as an outpatient in the hospital—reactions and side effects precautions.

Mary Ellen is on a new chemotherapy drug that is a monoclonal antibody. It helps her body have the capacity to fight the cancer. The name of the drug is Herceptin. It is a new variety of drug that works with the body's natural ability to sense cancer cells and discard them.

Checked into the hospital. Spent the day getting Herceptin infusion and Benadryl that left me sleepy. Found out why I was in the hospital. One of the side effects is anaphylactic shock. Whoa! Glad I didn't read that one ahead of time. I wondered why one nurse was with me the whole day and never left the room. Sometimes it pays not to read the fine print!

Now I'm on Herceptin/Taxotere cocktails or Herceptin straight up! Lots of bone pain.

M ary Ellen showed up today, Halloween, with a blue wig and broad-brimmed hat all covered with flowers and a butterfly. She wore a tan gingham raincoat. "Look! My hair grew back!" I love this woman's healthy sense of humor during this difficult time. I admire her, and we laugh. Today she was beginning to feel her energy draining and suspected her white blood cell count was low. From here she was en route to the doctor to get her blood count and begin the Neupogen injections, if necessary.

Mary Ellen is most comfortable lying on her back or her side, and so we worked together in one position, until there was a need to move. The left arm, mainly the underside, is still sensitive, so I tried to go lightly there with the touch and movement, but not with my intention. Sometimes when I came to those more sensitive areas, I found myself slowing down, as if honoring an unspoken request to really appreciate every detail of our interaction. Less playful, more supportive. Less inquiring what could be, more celebrating what is. Sometimes, Mary Ellen looked up with a painful expression and said or gestured that it was time for a pause. There are limits to movement. Sometimes this body needs a rest, a long moment to just be quiet and still.

I 'm back on Neupogen because of my blood counts. I can't remember things and my balance is affected. Sometimes I feel like I am staggering. I feel depressed and hopeless when I'm so sick.

Talked to my coach about being afraid. As always, he encouraged me to stay in the present. Above all, no fast forwarding or rewinding. I am not to be captivated by the past or the future. We talked about giving myself permission to do nothing.

My boys are fine. Mark is fine, because the Cardinals are in the playoffs. Michael is happily hiking in the English Lake District. Alleluia.

Did not go to my high school reunion, because my blood counts are so low. I was so exhausted; I didn't care. I have no energy at all. I am tired. When I feel so sick and am in this much pain, I feel I will not recover.
My CT scan shows something at the surgery site. They do not know what it is, so a PET scan is ordered. Is the cancer back already?

PET scan report confirms it is just a blobby thing. I can tell a lot by looking at medical people's eyes when they tell me things. I knew from the "get-go" that I had cancer, and that it was serious. I saw it in everyone's eyes. My oncologist did not have "the look" in his eyes when he told me about the blobby thing.

I had a massage today. During it, I remembered what it felt like to be able-bodied and well; it felt wonderful. I imagined my body like a beautiful garden in full bloom and humming with vibrant life. It was wonderful.

I am not feeling well. I am lonesome. My blood counts are down. I have to keep at this, and it feels almost impossible. I feel sick and exhausted all the time. Kitty and Finny are my companions today. They don't get tired of listening to me. It is all right with them if I cry. I love my cat and dog.

I understand now why people say they would rather die than take treatments. There is just so much you can face. Mom said she did not want treatment when she had her first diagnosis. But in the end, she did it.

X-rays, scanners, MRIs miss so much. They do not go deep enough. They do not get the whole picture. They cannot show images of thoughts, ideas, dreams, emotions, fear, desires, longings, and relationships.

It is so difficult to get to Mary. I feel sick. Right now I have to lean on her energy and positive thinking, because I have none.

Had a meltdown at the doc's. I told him I could not do this anymore. I said that the treatments were so difficult and that I was sick and tired of doing what everyone wearing a white coat told me to do. I was tired of being poked and jabbed and scanned. I was tired of being sick, and I was sick and tired of being sick and tired. I quit. He told me that I was like a marathon runner who had hit the wall. The end is not far off, but it is finishing the last piece that is so difficult. We agreed that I would take some time off and not have treatment during Thanksgiving week.

I find myself not standing up straight so I don't show my flat side.

THANKSGIVING

When I die,
I'd like to be buried on a lazy autumn afternoon
With the yawning sun basting the leaves
in deep reds, browns and yellows.
When the earth smells damp and rich,
And birds and squirrels clatter about,
Preparing for the frozen time ahead.
A languid laziness soothes my limbs
And blankets me in warmth
As I stretch contented in the autumn sun.
Death has touched me gently
With his long frosted fingers,
To remind me that one day he will return for good.
But, for now, I listen to the gentle drone of the bees,
Revel in the drift of swirling leaves,
And cherish the beauty of shadow and light.

© *Jan Newhouse, 2001.*

Mary Ellen came bringing a paperwhite bulb that she forced, happily announcing that she felt so much better. "This is my week off!" Mary Ellen reflected on how she went on strike last week. "I didn't do any exercises and wasn't pleasant. Instead, I just let all the built-up pain, impatience, and nastiness come out."

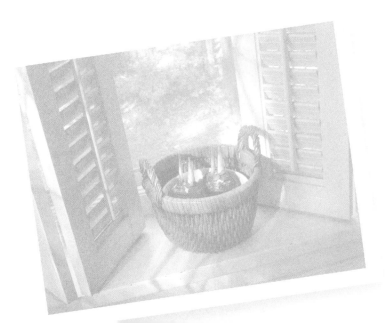

AUTUMN

*T*hank you note from Mary (that I keep beside my bed and read whenever I feel so sick):

> *I guess the paperwhite bulbs just put me over the top. Or maybe it's the Thanksgiving holiday. But there is just so much to be grateful for in you. Watching you bravely and authentically living through your cancer treatment has been a huge gift. I do sit in wonder at how you do it. How you continuously bring flowers, humor, costume, a good enough sense of being comfortable to show off incisions and grenades and share stories, and hugs. I hope this small reflection helps you pause and appreciate what a wonderful human being you are. Thank you for opening to love and being so alive. And thanks, too, for the beautiful paperwhites.*
>
> *Gratefully, Mary*

*M*ary Ellen was very chipper today. She had permission to skip one week of chemotherapy and so enjoyed a much more pleasant Thanksgiving. She said that her white blood cells were way up there yesterday when she went in for her chemotherapy.

Mary Ellen has been struggling with some of the arm exercises her surgeon taught her. "It's just not very comfortable on the underside of my left arm with certain movements." Still not ready for *Trager* movements here. However, her legs, right arm, and shoulders were very happy to stir around with me. Felt "wonderful, so much better," after the *Trager* work.

Winter

Today is my sister Rita's surprise fiftieth birthday. I do not feel well. I do not feel part of the family interaction. I like to sit and talk to my family members. The whole group is too much. I am so tired, I don't have the energy to pay attention.

People with hair have no idea how cold it is without hair. I was at a party recently and noticed a man wearing a hat inside the house. I knew immediately that he must be bald, although it was hard to tell given the style of his hat. We struck up a conversation and, sure enough, the reason for the hat was that he was bald and cold. We discussed baldness (among other things!) and shared our mutual experiences. Bald is cold.

Having a session with Mary with my bald head is a funny experience. When I had hair and I got my hair washed, I was familiar with the sound and the feel of someone running fingers through my hair. When Mary touches my bald head, there is no sound! And sometimes her hands are ice cold.

Mark is home from college. He looks wonderful. He came through the front door with his luggage, a big laundry basket full of dirty clothes! The look in Mark's eyes, when he saw me approach the front door, reminded me of the way all children look as they scan a group of adults and then, finally, find mom. I would see that look on his face when I picked him up at preschool and he spotted me.

     He had a great time in Minnesota with his Uncle John and Aunt Molly and his Iowa friends. Twenty-one days till Michael gets home. I am in a daze. I feel so much better after skipping that treatment. I need to speak up to those docs more often.

The snowstorm they predicted did arrive. I took a parking space close to the building today because, the way it was coming down, driving would soon become very difficult. People would cancel their plans, and the commerce in the building would slow way down, leaving plenty of spaces available. My office had that insulated feel that snow, building up

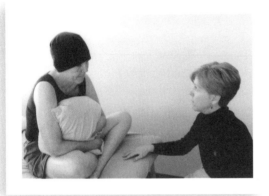

on rooftops and windowsills, gives. It was a day of waiting for the phone messages. Would anyone keep an appointment? The first three appointments canceled. Radio announcers were discouraging all from venturing out. A foot of snow was expected by mid afternoon.

At eleven o'clock Mary Ellen walked into the waiting room, dusting off snowflakes, transferring outer garments to the coat tree, and announcing that she had something to show me. Back in the treatment area, she pulled the new breast prosthesis and bra out of a bag. She has been fitted! She wanted me to handle the prosthesis and experience how realistic it feels, even the weight. Next she modeled her new ensemble to show me that she can reach behind her back to fasten the bra.

All this hoopla over new garments was a welcome distraction from the fact that she had had a chemotherapy treatment two days ago and that her arm was really hurting. She says that it is hard to extend her elbow, "like something won't give in there." The arm is most painful in the forearm, but the discomfort extends from shoulder to hand. Although talkative today, Mary Ellen did quiet at the end of the *Trager* session.

I had the best Christmas. I did not do one thing I did not want to do. I shopped in catalogs. I did not cook, clean, or preen. I simply enjoyed my family. We kept it simple, and it was great. We ate potluck at Cath's. Rita and Abby stayed here, and I was glad. I will remember this Christmas for a long time.

As our session closed today, Mary Ellen said, "What was coming to me today during *Trager* was that I feel strong and parts of me are very healthy, like my immune system. I haven't been sick the whole time I've been in treatment— knock on wood. Anyway, this feeling of being healthy is in sharp contrast to the experiences in the hospital and doctor's office. I am ready! My last dose of Herceptin is tomorrow. I'm ready to go!"

How can someone with a cancer diagnosis, undergoing treatment, tell me she hasn't been sick? What perspective did Mary Ellen have today during the *Trager* work? What feeling? What experience? What was larger and in sharper focus than the fatigue, nausea, and bone pain? What captured her mind in such a way as to provide this description of "not being sick" while in treatment?

Do I even need to know the details? Not really. Let this beautiful spirit of life come through!

I have my third Taxotere treatment tomorrow—no comment.

Had a session with Mary. She is such a help to me. She is a calming influence. She welcomes me into her office, where she has created a quiet, calm, peaceful space in a hurried and noisy world. While I am in that space I feel I am with someone who listens to my silence, my body, and my words. She is so respectful of my situation, so calm and unhurried. In many ways, Mary models what she teaches. She helps me rejoice in the body I have at this moment—to feel its strength, its movement. She helps me explore my earth space and my humanness. She and I have a spiritual connection during our sessions. She is not doing something to me. She and I are in a spiritual dance. Mary has helped me experience the body I have now and see that, while it is not the same, it is wonderful. She has seen all my grenades full of fluids of different colors and she does not cringe. All the preparation we did for surgery has helped me.

I am finished with chemo, and in a strange way, I wish I weren't. At least we were doing something. Every ache and pain is cancer returning. I feel very edgy, as if all my nerve endings are exposed. I am tired all the time.

I want to do so much with my boys, but I am so tired.

Who is the new Mary Ellen? I feel her beginning to emerge.

I went to the symphony hairless, hatless, and happy!

Cancer has reminded me of the importance of bowing. When I was in the convent, we did a certain amount of bowing. We bowed when entering and leaving the choir, the refectory, when passing Mother Superior. Bowing was an expression of humility and reverence. I like bowing. There is a certain acknowledgment that I am not the center of it all, and that I have a lot to learn. Cancer is reminding me how to bow. Each day I have something new to learn. Each person I meet has something to teach me. I bow before it all, the beauty of the world, the wonder of creation, the majesty of the universe, the power of love.

Oh God, thank you for my being and for my being here.

Mary Ellen has finished receiving the Taxotere treatments—Hallelujah! But she must continue taking the Herceptin for an undetermined time, which is related to tumor markers and other things. With chemotherapy coming to an end, Mary Ellen's life has begun to take on some semblance of normalcy. She went swimming today for the first time since last April. I felt better just knowing Mary Ellen had been back in her beloved pool! She told me she'll spend a long weekend with women from the parish at Cedar Creek and is looking forward to it—everything but the 10,000 questions.

Mary Ellen was over the slight cold she had last week. Because her blood counts have been low, she's been taking antibiotics. Today Mary Ellen insisted that *Trager* should be done in the water. She was happy to report that the self-massage of the arm really helped. She said she finds that the area of sensitivity diminishes with massage—that she can rest her upper arm on the sheet, and it is not uncomfortable. How happy Mary Ellen was to show me the ease of reaching her arm overhead.

A lot of laughter, about warm hands, crones, global warming, queens, etc., punctuated our session today.

Mary Ellen has seen the lymphedema doctor and knows "everything you can know about lymphedema without going to medical school."

She said the *Trager* moves under her shoulder felt like the image of being surrounded by her friends in the surgical suite. She's using the imagery tape to prepare for radiation.

I find that I now feel able to return to the common shower at the pool. My friends are great, and one even said she had been wondering when I was going to stop showering with my left arm covering my surgery site. Then, today, for the first time, the high school girls' soccer team decided to use the showers during the early morning swimmers' time. There I was standing, bald-headed, one breasted, and saying "Hi" to my son's friends! Later I told my son about it. His response was to say that he had never been so embarrassed in his life! He was embarrassed?!

Mary Ellen looked darling in her Art Fair hat. There's really no hint of baldness when she has it on. This is a classy look, a soft, black felt with just the right amount of fabric rose adorning the crown.

Mary Ellen recounted to me that last night, while lying in bed worrying about her son, she thought to herself, "let go of the worry." Immediately, she felt her right shoulder muscles release.

Mary Ellen can taste food a little bit again. She noticed it while eating a hard-boiled egg.

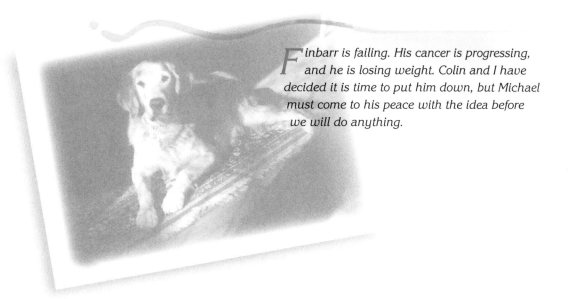

Finbarr is failing. His cancer is progressing, and he is losing weight. Colin and I have decided it is time to put him down, but Michael must come to his peace with the idea before we will do anything.

WINTER

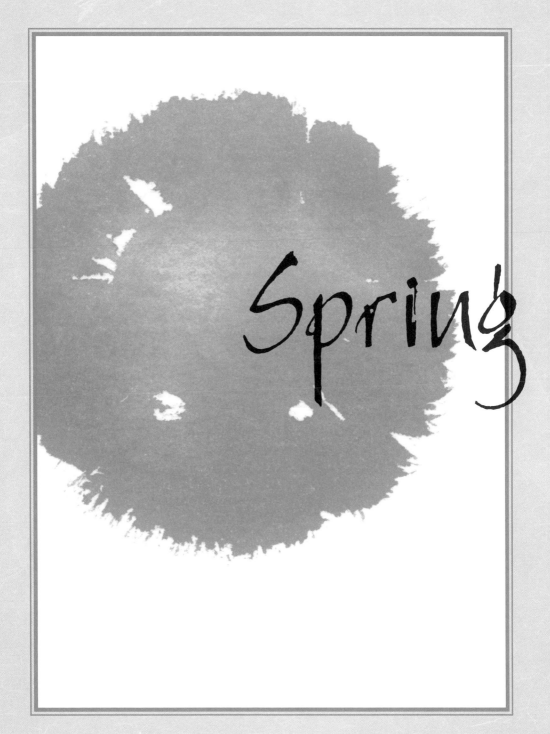

Spring

Mary Ellen reminded me that it has almost been a year since her diagnosis. She asked the oncologist if he thought she had to begin radiation March 16 as planned, because she wants to go out of town March 17 for a week. He said he thought it would be OK to wait. That means she won't begin until March 28. She'll go daily for 6 weeks and be finished just a few days after Easter. She remembered that the oncologist told her at the time of diagnosis, "You have an opportunity, now." She became teary thinking of this. Mary Ellen reflected on how cancer changes you... on how she has tried to be present to it, to participate in her own healing, and how she has taken the opportunity given to her. She talked about some of the loneliness, of being so uncomfortable in the middle of the night with the chemo. Mary Ellen continues to remind me of my "crone power," experienced through the warmth and energy of my hands. She also continues to remind me to take some days off. "How many people have you disappointed today?"

Smiling as usual, but with fear just underneath the surface, Mary Ellen told me she is scared to death, because she has had pain over the left ribs since Saturday. She was reaching and heard something pop, then felt a warmth in the area where the pain is now. Nothing became painful until later. But all she can think of is that the cancer is spreading, and it's all through her thorax and what if, after all of this, she dies?

Tears. We agreed that she would lie on her back while I applied the vitamin E to the skin of the chest and things settled down a little. This worked well. Felt better. "Can you tell if a certain structure is strained?" "Yes." We looked at the anatomy book together, then I palpated the cartilage of the 9th, 10th, and 11th ribs. That's exactly where she was most tender. I asked Mary Ellen if deep breathing reproduced the pain. "Yes." I tied a big sheet around Mary Ellen while she was seated to support her thorax, and this gave immediate relief. "Well, it's probably just musculoskeletal pain," I surmised, "but please report it to your doctor." I encouraged her to use a corset at home, a heating pad off and on, and to take deep breaths.

For a lot of this session we talked about the movie *Chocolat* and how much we both enjoyed it. She looked more reassured at the end.

I went to see Lisa to show her that my head is now covered with fuzz. I sat in her hairdressing chair, covered myself with a drape, and told her I would close my eyes and she could give me a whole new hairstyle— a complete makeover! She combed and brushed and used the blow dryer as customers walked by, and we had the best laughs.

"It feels so good to feel good. It gives me so much hope." Mary Ellen is in a small hiatus of treatment, between the end of chemo and the beginning of radiation. She conversed today about being on a committee overseeing the renovation of her church. The contrast between dealing with the worries of cancer and dealing with the complaints of parishioners is laughable! Her ribs feel almost back to normal.

I drove to Miniwanca with Michael for a few days. I cannot quite believe I am actually here. I am exhausted and in pain all the time, but I am here. I made it! I will talk to the director while I am here about working for the American Youth Foundation. This is part of my recovery. Oh God, thank you for my being and for my being here. It is truly a wonderful time when Michael and I drive home together from Miniwanca. We talk a lot, and we are quiet a lot. We have such a special relationship: our mutual love of the dunes and Lake Michigan and all that is so magical about Miniwanca.

I have a simulation tomorrow of my upcoming radiation treatment—and then radiation all week. I am almost finished with the treatment plan set out over a year ago. This has been such a year of grace for me.

Because it is important to radiate me in the same area every day for six weeks, I had a custom body mold made! I have to hold my left arm over my head during the treatment, and that is hard for me. Then they use computers and lasers to see that I am in the right position for radiating the areas that are drawn all over my chest and neck. I have "my map to wellness" drawn right on me.

Most people do not invite guests into their homes and then go to the basement (unless, of course, it is a finished basement). No, one usually does not go to the dingy basement—all battleship gray in chipped paint—and sit under the exposed pipes and wires. The ceilings are not as high in the basement as in the rest of the house. Most people like to sit near windows, if not for the fresh air, at least for the light, and most basements are windowless. In addition, most basements are damp. I have just described the area of the hospital where I have radiation each day!

Never go to radiation without a friend.

Having a session with Mary is so different from going to some docs for treatment. The docs tell me how sick I am and how much treatment they know I need. With Mary I come to feel well, and I am treated as though I know what I need and what would be good for me. We work on the treatment together. Dancing again!

Found out that Mary Ellen drove to Miniwanca last weekend (a trip of about 500 miles.) "Hey! You don't have cancer. You're not sick!" I had to tease. There is more to the story. After arriving home and checking voice mail, her own voice was on the answering machine, calling from somewhere in northern Illinois, saying she was doing fine and just checking in. But, upon hearing it, she did not remember making the call!

"Well, there it is. Another example of 'chemobrain,'" she said. I listened to her story about memory loss and thought about how I have noticed she needs to be reminded of certain routines now, such as scheduling the next appointment or writing the check for the session. The memory loss is expected during chemotherapy treatment and expected to resolve after chemotherapy is over. I am trusting that this is true. I am imagining the day Mary Ellen's memory is reliable again and how her youthfulness will seem to reappear.

Mary Ellen had been to radiation today for the first time. Just the way she likes to call the warm massage table "a warm rock," the mold

In Colin's Words

When what is billed as the last stage of breast cancer treatment—radiology—is beginning, I find my role is starting to change. Mary Ellen received chemotherapy treatment on a three-week cycle, and I had made an arrangement with my office that enabled me to accompany her to each treatment. Now radiation is going to be applied on a daily basis, and it is necessary for me to hand over to the rest of her "team" the task of accompanying her to each daily session after the first.

I have, as a result, the opportunity to anticipate by a few weeks and to a small degree the feeling of letdown that Mary Ellen can expect when her treatment ends. Although the year of supporting and sharing breast cancer with her has been full of fear and the sense of panic that comes with helplessness, the medical regimen and the measured series of procedures brought with them a sense of comfort. They answered the question, "What do we do next?" and they limited the horizon to a manageable length of time. When she finishes her last radiation, all that is going to change. She is going to be left asking, "Has it all worked?" and also left with a self-imposed feeling of obligation to get back to normal. At the selfish level, I am feeling exhausted and yet I know that in many ways my cheerleading job is far from over. I have been with her when the oncologist has explained that the tumor marker in her remained steady since the mastectomy, and I know that is good news. I know, too, how strong she really is and that she will weather the future as she has weathered the past. It is just that I love her so much and want her to be well and whole, and I want to *know* that she is well and whole. ●

she had to have made for radiation was also warm, and so a positive association was made.

Today, during *Trager* she described how, when she feels her right shoulder creeping up or the left hand clenching something, she'll say, "Why am I doing this?" And let go. "You taught me this," she said a couple of times today. She asked, "Well, how far down does a shoulder go?" and imagined warm taffy being stretched. "You taught me this," she said. She remarked that during her early experiences of *Trager,* when I first came under her upper back with my hands and lifted, she thought, "This is what it must be like to be a baby!"

I have to do such preparation in order to get myself to the radiation area each day. The claustrophobia comes with me. So I am so glad that the door is not visible from the radiation area. I am certain that they have left it open a crack.

I am in awe of the people I meet at radiation. Some are so obviously ill and yet so brave and determined to do what will help them. Others are very quiet, but I have started a little conversation each day and pretty soon others join in and we break the fearful and lonely silence in the only way we know how. We laugh and talk about our situations. But we are very careful never to ask too many questions, because I do not think any of us wants to know the whole truth of another's diagnosis. This is so because we all want to hold onto our own hope and not have it shattered, at least not here.

I have asked Mary to apply Vitamin E to the radiation area. We have done this both in preparation for the radiation and now that it is in progress. I wonder how my ribs and heart are doing. They have lost the protective covering of my breast and are exposed to all that radiation.

Radiation seems like such an innocuous procedure. I lie in a mold. The technical people all leave the room and communicate via microphone and TV monitor. Machines whirr and move all around me. I get up and go home. But I am in a lead-lined room with a door the size and thickness of a bank vault door. This is powerful stuff. No wonder I am concerned about my ribs and heart.

My antidote to all of this is a session with Mary. Lots of windows, soft light, quiet, one medical person, laughter, peace, stories.

The opener today was Mary Ellen lifting up her shirt in front of the mirror, exposing the blue and orange lines criss-crossing her chest and proceeding to point to each, naming them for the highways that one takes to Camp Miniwanca, one of her favorite places in the whole world. There's the map, right on her chest!

She told me she has had radiation daily for a week and explained that once she is in the mold, she is further positioned by the use of lasers shot across her. It's scary to know that people leave the room completely for the few minutes she is there being radiated. So, she imagines that the door is left open a crack.

Because of the outline on her chest, Mary Ellen was very worried that her heart was being radiated. The doctors explained that the part of her heart that was being affected was the size of her fingernail and that the rays come into her from the side, not the top. This was a great relief. During the *Trager* work today, Mary Ellen exclaimed how good it feels to be in her body. "My body just feels so good!" Part of this stems from the left arm feeling better. The lymphedema has improved. The swimming and other exercises have improved the flexibility. The left arm really liked being handled just the way the right arm was. The leg movements reminded her of being in the water.

Mary Ellen has taught me a lot about how to respond in an artful, human way to what life presents. How clever, in recognizing her discomfort of being alone in the radiation lab, to simply imagine the door being left open a crack. A connection with the others was thus maintained. And, instead of wallowing in negative self-judgment about the look of blue and orange marker lines across her chest, she instead sees the map to her beloved Miniwanca. Of course, the map is right there, over her heart.

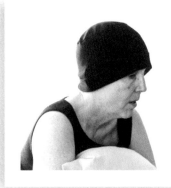

When the technicians leave me in the room for my radiation treatments, I sometimes start to cry. I cry out of fear—fear that my heart is being damaged, fear about this scary procedure, but also because sometimes a good rinse is necessary, and so I just spend some time rinsing.

There is a man at radiation who likes crossword puzzles. He is always reading, and I am sometimes doing a puzzle. He noticed me doing puzzles and asked if I was stuck. So we struck up a conversation about crossword puzzles, and other things just followed. He is quiet and somewhat shy. One day he introduced me to his son and his wife. I found out that he is a retired physician (I've noticed that there are a lot of retired docs in radiation). We just clicked. That is all I know about him. Then on a recent visit he told me that he was finished with his treatments and would not be coming back. I told him that I would miss him. Then he said that he wished he had some of my spirit. I told him he could have as much as he needed, whenever he needed it.

I was aware of having an infection just beginning in my scratchy throat and had given Mary Ellen the option over the phone to skip today's visit. But she said, if I wore a mask, she would be fine. So there we were. I was wearing a mask, and she is hard of hearing in the left ear. It was most comical. The clear sound of the words in my head, before I spoke them, was ambushed by the mask. Their utterance bore no resemblance to my intention. I burst with laughter, partly from Mary Ellen's puzzled expression, partly from the mumble that tumbled forth. Ahem. Collecting my composure I tried again, thinking a slower pace and better enunciation would help. Mary Ellen still couldn't play back an intelligible sentence. Laughter again. Finally, "let me stand by your good ear."

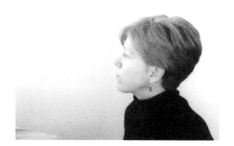

"Yes, that helps. We can do this!" We staved off the spread of infection and had no idea it would be so much fun!

In our continuing ritual of choosing a Wisdom Card at the beginning of each meeting, Mary Ellen and I did so again today. For the first time, we each picked a card that had a similar message and the message was forgiveness.

"I have the power to make changes. It is so comfortable to play victim, because it is always someone else's fault. I have to stand on my own two feet and take some responsibility."

*"I am centered in truth and peace. I search my heart for injustices
I still harbor. I forgive them and let them go."*

This was also the first session during which Mary Ellen went into a very
deep state of relaxation. She was very still, with small muscular movements happening occasionally in the hands and feet. I was speaking
to her after the hands-on work was completed and didn't get the usual
immediate response. Then all of a sudden, her eyes flew open and she
said, "Where did I go? I thought you were my sister!"

*I have never fallen asleep in a session with Mary. But it really wasn't
sleep… I went somewhere. But I don't know where I went. I think it
has to do with trust. I have always found real trust of another difficult,
and there I was trusting. There is, it seems to me, a dance in a* Trager
*session. Mary and I are caught up in a dance. We are human beings
connected in a unique way to each other's souls and, for a brief
moment, we experience connection and trust through movement,
a spiritual movement.*

*My cousin was buried yesterday. How does a family deal with losing
him so tragically? No one can make sense out of this, and I suppose
we never will. But I went to the cemetery where many members of my
family are buried in order to make peace with my past. I do not need to
live up to anyone's expectations, to be someone I am not. Now is the
time to tell the truth, to be honest, to let go, and to be grateful for what
they gave me.*

*Today I asked Mary what she thought about when she was moving
my feet and legs. I asked her if she made her grocery list. She told me
that, ideally, she thinks about nothing. Throughout this year I have
spent a lot of time thinking about nothing. I call it staying in the present
moment. I guess it is the same thing.*

Referring to her cancer treatment experience, Mary Ellen had another
great line today: "I've been poisoned, slashed, and burned! No, make
that, I've been poisoned, slashed, poisoned, and burned!"

At the beginning of the *Trager* work today, Mary Ellen sat up on the massage table and asked me what I was thinking about while I was practicing *Trager*. Was I making a grocery list in my head? I explained that I was intending to be present in the moment as much as possible and that I am not present in the moment all the time. She responded that she thought she could tell that sometimes I was not present. Then she remarked that *Trager* is a dance, that there is a real moment-by-moment communication going on between the two people. I responded that this is true and that not everyone can dance as well as she can.

The *Trager* continued and I noticed today that her neck movements were really freer than they have been in recent memory. It is the kind of freedom of movement that draws me deeper into the experience. It was a luscious feeling, this movement that just flowed so effortlessly in my hands. The cervical vertebrae seemed to be floating in a soft, but elastic, wrapping.

Later, in processing the session, Mary Ellen told me that, while I was working with her head and neck, she saw a very bright light. She opened her eyes briefly, thinking she would see the sun beaming in through the window, but it was darker in the room when her eyes were open than when her eyes were shut. So she closed her eyes again and, in fact, the bright light was still there. She said it was her healing light.

We confirm with words our deep connection: her bright light, my awareness of a greater freedom in the neck movements. Gratitude wells up in me, and I bow to the Healer's presence.

On my way to radiation today, we were stopped at a red light, when a tractor-trailer moved left to right through the intersection in front of us. It was unusual in that it was painted all over in the style of a Monet painting. There was a beautiful pastoral scene including ladies with parasols walking through the countryside. I immediately thought it must be some sort of an ad for the art museum. But there was no writing on the side of the truck facing me. It was only when I saw the end of the truck as it drove through the intersection that I read that it was actually a mobile mammography truck, I guess on its way to a "location near you." My reaction was not the one that the sponsors of that truck intended, I am sure. It is difficult for me to look at the prettifying of cancer. Cancer and its treatment—the chemotherapy, the fear, the exhaustion, the pain, the drugs, the isolation, the disfiguring surgery—

are not beautiful. That truck should have said, "STOP EVERYTHING AND GET IN HERE AND SAVE YOUR LIFE," in the biggest, boldest, darkest letters they could find. It should have had a siren on top making all the noise possible. I wonder, if that truck had held a screening device for prostate cancer, how it would have been decorated. While I understand the notion of the pink ribbons worn by so many— including my oncologist—and all the pink jewelry, I don't like them. They are examples of the prettifying of cancer. Pink is wimpy, not the color needed to deal with this disease. Pink is Barbie's color. Why do we have to make reminders of cancer cute and soft and pink when, in reality, it is nothing like that?

We put Finny down today. Michael stayed home from school for Fin's last day. We took him to Forest Park and carried him to the waterfall so he could lie next to the water he so loved. We sat and enjoyed the sights, the sounds, and the smells. Colin, Michael, and I held him as the doctor injected him and he died. He was such a fantastic dog.

I miss Finbarr so much.

I sometimes wonder whether it really matters if I am physically healed. I am not sure that that is the issue. Inner life, spiritual life, is also important. Healing somehow involves letting go—letting go of expectations, shoulds, anger, resentment, guilt. Sometimes I wonder if there is a part of me that fears getting well. After all, I am the focus of lots of attention. I've stopped working outside my home during the treatments. Not much is expected of me. I am actually off the speeding treadmill. When I wake up in the morning, I notice that the awful dread I experienced before this diagnosis is gone, the dread that used to accompany mornings when I did not want to get out of bed and face the day. My cell phone is not interrupting meetings. I do not have long "to do" lists. Those lists meant I was needed. I was important. I was necessary. I could point to all that I had accomplished by all the things I had checked off my lists. If I am working hard, have long lists, am always tired, always behind, then I must be good. Then maybe I will be loved. For the first time in my life, I feel comfortable saying "no." When I do not go to book club, church, work, meetings, family gatherings, my excuse is air tight, "I'm sick."

I know getting well means I must make changes. I must practice saying no and disappointing people. I need to grow up on the inside and stop playing the child in relationships and choices. Children always have someone else to blame. Children always make excuses. Growing up means looking inside honestly and facing my personal inner truths. Going to doctors can be addictive. Lots of attention, sympathy. What's not to like? Getting well means growing up and breaking old addictions.

Mastectomy is a disfiguring surgery. I am bothered by having to wear a prosthesis all the time, if I want to look "normal." Who am I looking normal for? What the heck is normal? Is anyone really looking? Does it matter?

I no longer have an active real estate license. Another piece of the recovery is in order.

What am I going to do about a bathing suit? That will be really weird trying to swim with some foreign object stuck to my chest. Then, when I get out of the water, I'll have to wring out one side of my chest! Maybe this prosthesis will pop up out of the water, as I am swimming, and land on my shoulder! Maybe I'll just use it as a flotation device instead of a kickboard. It is a good thing I have lots of friends at the pool.

It's early May, more than a year from the day Mary Ellen first came in asking for the support of the *Trager* Approach in her cancer treatment. She told me she has begun getting her "boost," which is extra radiation that will last a week. "My sentence has been lengthened." Even so, she appears to be in pretty good spirits.

Mary Ellen told me that, while lying in the mold surrounded by all the high-tech radiation equipment, she has been asking, "What can be easier, softer, lighter?" She said it helps her recall the bodily ease she has become acquainted with here in our sessions together. Then, the times of her radiation treatment, still lonely and frightening, aren't just something to endure but an opportunity to remember how relaxed and comfortable she can be. She also imagines the laser lights as healing lights. I admire her active participation in her own healing. This is the truth. This is what we are all capable of doing, cultivating an attitude of receptivity and deepening our awareness of how we are a powerful force in the overall process of getting well.

The skin on the left side of Mary Ellen's upper back looked a little sunburned. At her request, I took time to apply the Aquaphore, which is very soothing. Today, I was almost heavy with the collective remembrance of the trauma this dear body has been through. And it made me feel lucky. Not in a glad-it-wasn't-me sort of way. No, it made me feel lucky to be here—knowing this person, being the one who can touch with a message of hopeful expectation. And more than that. Being the one who has the privilege to witness. Being the one who gets to be with this person of faith.

The mood of the *Trager* session today was holy. My mood? Perhaps. The body is honored by the touch of every limb, the belly and chest, the head and neck. I noticed a deeper calm in the way Mary Ellen lay on the table today. It was mostly something I sensed on a gut level, but my eye scanned for some confirming visual information. No wrinkles of facial expression. Her breathing reminded me of sleep. I paused in the moment, inundated by a sense of my own great fortune.

Shifting back to the room, Mary Ellen appeared almost alarmed to have been quieted so deeply. I reassured her in her half upright position and she lay back down. I reminded her to pause, then move slowly and gently off the table as she felt ready.

Looking over to the counter of the sink, I noticed the Ziplock bag of sand from Miniwanca that Mary Ellen brought here today. She has offered to make me a mini-sandbox for my office.

*M*ark comes home tomorrow. Freshman year is over.

I have noticed in sessions with Mary that my muscles have memory. I wonder if that is the same thing as noses having memory. Whenever I smell carnations, I am reminded of high school dances and corsages, and I immediately smile. My ears have memory in that, whenever I listen to Pavarotti sing "Nessun Dorma," I am with mom and I weep just the way we both did when we listened to it together. We both adored it so. Maybe muscles and tissues are the same way. Remembering through them what it feels like to be caressed, carried, protected, soothed, rocked, cherished—these are all memories carried in my muscles and tissues.

Great bumper sticker: What if the hokey pokey is what it's all about?

I am changing my mind about healing. I always thought that, if I wanted to be healed, I had to find a healer. But I understand now that the patient is the healer as well. The doctors are the technical side of the equation. Very necessary. Then there is the spiritual side. Very necessary. But the sick person must be willing to make the necessary life changes. These include changing old unhealthy habits, forgiving old grudges, letting go of old wounds. The real healer is the patient, when ready.

Habits of a lifetime that have not served me well must be given up, including the old time-honored excuse "that's just the way I am." Then there is the fact of disappointing lots of people, because it is time I stick up for myself.

DIRECTIONS
Do not try to rescue the driftwood.
Let the sand scour its surface
And the waves wash it clean.

Wait for the storm to subside.
Listen to the gentling of the waves.
Finger the smoothness of the wood.
This is your legacy.

© *Jan Newhouse, 2000.*

Mary Ellen told me a lot of things today that are fundamental *Trager* philosophies. First she told me stories of "recall," lying in bed at night, remembering what it is like to be here, remembering on a feeling level. This has helped her to relax, to become more comfortable and go to sleep. Secondly, she told me about being aware of her whole body, not just the part that is being treated or is uncomfortable. There is so much of her that feels good. Thirdly, she told me a story of lying in the radiation mold and having to be so still and to be postured just so and how she has discovered that she can lift just one finger and notice how easy that is. Then to lift it again and imagine what could be easier than that.

As we began the hands-on work, there were visible burns on the skin of the chest and also the shoulder area. Therefore, I was unable to handle Mary Ellen as casually in *Trager* as is usually possible. I'll wait to be able to fully touch the left upper body. Mary Ellen said, "It would be nice if the upper half felt as good as the lower half." This was a talkative session and, at a certain point, we both acknowledged that we couldn't talk and fully enter into the *Trager* experience. From my vantage point today, the movement of the right scapula was especially wavelike, as I came underneath her with both hands as she lay on her back. We were amazed by this, and we talked about it afterward.

There are docs and medical professionals who get it. I have met them.

> *Their egos are out of the picture.*
> *They are open-hearted.*
> *They want healthy patients, not credit.*
> *They understand that medicine is an art as well as a science.*
> *They are compassionate.*
> *They understand that the body, though broken, houses a spirit that wants to be well.*
> *They realize that one can be healed and still die.*
> *They focus on the parts of the body that are well.*
> *They do not see disease sitting on the table in a paper gown.*
> *They have a sense of humor.*
> *They do not take themselves too seriously.*
> *They are aware that healing comes from within.*
> *They realize that health and illness are mysteries and that illness is more than a set of symptoms.*
> *They love their patients.*
> *They realize that they must accompany their patients on the path to healing.*
> *They encourage their patients to enter into the spiritual side of healing.*

Mary Ellen was so taken with the sky today that she pulled the blinds all the way up on the middle window of my office and had me look up and out. It was a gorgeous sky, the kind you sail under or mountain climb into. We repositioned the table a little so she could have her head next to the window and just watch the sky. If this wasn't distraction enough, the rest of our time together was punctuated with interruptions. Staying present in the body and focused was a bit of a challenge when first, the electricity went out, signaled by a beep from the window AC unit. There were a couple of more beeps until the electricity finally came back on. Then there was a shout from outside my office door, so I had to check and see if there was a UPS delivery. As we resumed the *Trager*, a storm began blowing in very hard, making loud gusty sounds. Moments later a fire engine and emergency vehicle drove up, sirens blaring. They stopped just below our window, at the lobby entrance to the building.

Finding myself distracted, I half expected Mary Ellen to pop open an eye and poke fun at the series of events. But instead, she lay quietly, taking an occasional deep breath. I know it is possible to have such focused attention, but for some reason, witnessing Mary Ellen's example, it seemed all new to me.

Last session. Mary Ellen had her scans and she is free of cancer. Free of cancer. She will be going to Miniwanca this weekend.

The Wisdom Card today said:

Healing means to make whole and to accept all parts of myself—
not just the parts I like, but all of me. I can heal myself on all levels.

As Mary Ellen read this out loud, it summed up so much. Her eyes were so clear and filled with truth as she looked at me, and we sat in the silence of that wisdom.

I don't remember so much about the details of the *Trager* session today. I do remember being in a rarefied space. Free of cancer. She had come out on the other side. This is a milestone, a new beginning. A sense of mystery enveloped me and us. There is another chance. It could have turned out a million different ways. It turned out this way.

The farewell hug was full of recognition of our teamwork, of gratitude for the moment, and for each other.

As she walked out the door Mary Ellen turned and said, "You go, too, with all your healing and holy work that you do here in this room."

I am experiencing some withdrawal symptoms now that treatment is over. The process of cancer treatment involved regimentation. It provided me with a schedule and something for me to do. Now that it has ended, I feel I have lost a certain amount of control. I was focused, and now there is a big let down. I find myself imagining that the people I meet assume that, because I look physically better, I must be feeling well. They must be thinking, "Why doesn't she just snap out of it?"

As I look back and think about my relationships with my caregivers, it seems that I had a need to invest them with a degree of caring that was superhuman. Making them all-knowing and all-caring gave me something at the time that was very meaningful. Now, from a different perspective, I can see them as real people with real feelings and be glad about it. I think I spent a number of years doing something very similar to God. The God I knew was the God I needed.

The other day I yelled out, "Has anyone seen my breast?" We were getting ready to go out, and I could not find it. Colin came into our room, and we found it at the foot of our bed. I had somehow made the bed over the prosthesis. When it fell on the floor I said, "Whatever you do, don't step on my breast." We've come a long way! I live each day with a companion called chronic disease. I know it is there. I have learned so much from it. My health is now a part of my decision making, what I eat, what I choose to do, where I choose to go, the people I choose to be with. Cancer has been my teacher, and I continue to learn from it. It has taught me that it is

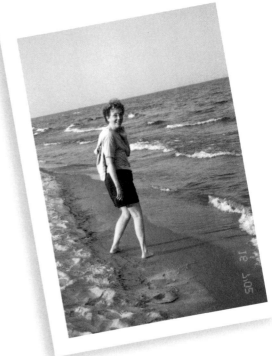

important just to be, to live in the present moment, to breathe and, above all, to be grateful. It has taught me that peace comes not from getting what I want but from ceasing to be unhappy with what is there. Cancer is teaching my heart to dance!

"Genuine healing is a journey, facilitated by a healer, into a broken and hurt self, the purpose of which is to encounter a depth of humanity deeper than the tragedy of any illness. The healer takes a person into the disorder and brokenness, whether it is curable or incurable, to find an intactness and reconciliation that profoundly reflects and manifests the genuine self.

Healing is a crucible to encounter the source of our being in our worst times; it is our genuine and potentially intact response to chaos, anguish, and suffering. Healers forge the illness, the techniques, and their special healing relationship into an opportunity to uncover the truth of who we really are.

Healing is not something we do only when we are sick; it is part of the process and journey of life."

TED KAPTCHUK
HEALERS ON HEALING

APPENDIX: SOURCES

1. Achterburg, Jeanne. *Imagery in Healing: Shamanism and modern medicine.* Boston: New Science Library, an imprint of Shambala Publications Inc., 1985.

2. Guided Imagery Tapes
    Image Paths, Inc.
    P.O. Box 5714
    Cleveland, OH 44101
    (800) 800-8661
    Copyright © 1993 Time Warner Audiobooks, a Time Warner Company, 9229 Sunset Blvd., Los Angeles, CA 90069.

3. Wisdom Cards
    Louise L. Hay
    Hay House, Inc.
    P.O. Box 5100
    Carlsbad, CA 92018-5100
    (800) 654-5126
    Web site: www.hayhouse.com
    Copyright © 2000 by Hay House, Inc. Reprinted by permission of Hay House, Inc.

4. Carlson, Richard and Shield, Benjamin (Eds.). *Healers on Healing.* Los Angeles: Jeremy P. Tarcher, 1989.

5. Huddleston, Peggy. *Prepare for Surgery, Heal Faster: A guide of mind-body techniques.* Cambridge, MA: Angel River Press, 1996.

6. Newhouse, Jan. Unpublished poems. "Directions," © 2000; "Into the Valley of the Shadow," © 2000; "Thanksgiving," © 2001. Poems reprinted by permission of Jan Newhouse.

7. *2002 Nursing Drug Handbook,* 22nd edition. Springhouse, PA: Springhouse Corporation, 2002.

8. Rinpoche, Sogyal. *The Tibetan Book of Living and Dying.* New York: HarperCollins Publishers, 1993.

For additional information about *Trager*®

9. Juhan, Deane. *Job's Body: A handbook for bodywork* (2nd ed.). Barrytown, New York: Barrytown, Ltd., 1998.
   E-mail: publishers@stationhill.org
   Web site: www.stationhill.org

10. Liskin, Jack. *Moving Medicine: The life and work of Milton Trager, M.D.* Barrytown, NY: Station Hill Press, 1996.

11. Trager, Milton with Guadagno-Hammond, Cathy. *Trager Mentastics: Movement as a way to agelessness.* Barrytown, NY: Station Hill Press, 1987.

12. Trager International
    24800 Chagrin Blvd., Suite 205
    Beachwood, OH 44122
    (216) 896-9383
    E-mail: admin@trager.com
    Web site: www.trager.org

13. United States Trager Association
    24800 Chagrin Blvd., Suite 205
    Beachwood, OH 44122
    (216) 896-9383
    E-mail: admin@trager-us.org
    Web site: www.trager-us.org